the *smart* girl's
guide to porn

the *smart* girl's guide to porn

Violet Blue

CLEIS
PRESS

Published in the United States by Cleis Press Inc.,
P.O. Box 14697, San Francisco, California 94114.

Printed in the United States.
Cover design: Scott Idleman
Cover photograph: Sylvie Blum
Book design: Karen Quigg
Cleis Press logo art: Juana Alicia
First Edition.
10 9 8 7 6 5 4 3 2 1

Library of Congress Cataloging-in-Publication Data

Blue, Violet.
The smart girl's guide to porn / Violet Blue. — 1st ed.
        p. cm.
     ISBN-13: 978-1-57344-247-3 (pbk. : alk. paper)
     ISBN-10: 1-57344-247-X (pbk. : alk. paper)
1. Pornography. 2. Sex instruction for women. 3. Sexual
   excitement. I. Title.
     HQ471.B643 2006
     613.9'6—dc22   2006014862

Contents

introduction: the smart girls' porn club

I have a confession to make: I never went to journalism school to become a porn critic. While I'd had a few experiments with boyfriends and made some hasty rental decisions, with mixed results, I hadn't really thought of porn as being something that one would evaluate in a critical context, as in good vs. bad. Much like the words *smart phone* and *comfortable flight*, the concept of putting the words *good* and *porn* together in one meaningful sentence seemed like a contradiction of terms. One thing is for sure. when they asked me to become a porn reviewer at my job eight years ago, I jumped at the chance because it gave me the opportunity to watch porn for a living.

I wasn't picked for the job because I like going to work in my bunny slippers. Nor even because I like porn. (I do.) No one knows for sure how one becomes a pro-porn pundit and female porn reviewer, but one thing's for certain: I do it because I enjoy explicit sexual imagery. When it's good, it turns me on. And I've learned over the years that an awful lot of women are like me in that respect. Despite what anyone says about women and porn, the truth is that many of us look at it for one very good reason: because we like to.

But, of course, usually pornography isn't very good. I remember the first time I had a feeling of porn hope. It came one minute before porn dismay. You know, the wish to see something hot, and not scary or disappointing. I wasn't a total novice before I started work as a porn reviewer: I knew about porn. I had watched a few videos before with boyfriends. Either they themselves rented and brought the tapes home, or together we sauntered through the western-style adults only swinging doors and did our best to make out the promise of the tiny pictures on the box covers, looking for even a scrap of what we hoped to see. And no matter what, when we got all set in front of the TV with lube in hand, the videos were bad. Really bad. Worse than after-school specials, worse than community theater; more like The Weather Channel. Which, last time I checked, is hot for only a small segment of the population.

My first real porn hope came when I browsed a porn catalog that I bought for a dollar at a local women-run sex toy store. The shop sported a colorful paint job and displayed handwritten reviews of erotic books and vibrators, and possessed a reputation as a women-friendly place to peruse and buy sex gear. I was intrigued by and often visited its many racks of adult videos, but hadn't brought anything home. Still, the store beckoned to me as my brave new world, full of promise and excitement. Its catalog whispered a promise to my libido: its contents were supposedly videos handpicked by cultured, sex-happy female reviewers. They promised to be savvy selections by women like me, or at least women who hired punk chicks who could sell me a vibrator and a catalog with a smile and a wink. The store featured porn directed by women, ostensibly created for women viewers. The catalog fed my fantasies of better sex—a better life!—with videos described as having "high production values," "excellent plot," and "good-natured, unrestrained sex fests." It left me believing that with a little guidance, porn could be good.

They only tricked me a few times. I brought home tape after tape of grunting and sweating porn performers, and though once in a while I caught a glimpse of sexuality that turned my crank, their cornucopias of cartoonish porn stars, overstuffed and underfed starlets, and soft-focus feminist porn clearly didn't portray the type of sex that girls like me were actually having. Or, at least, wanted to have. Or just wanted to see others having. Everything looked like it was from the 1980s—even the brand-new titles, and most especially the sex acts. No one had ever told me what to think about porn before this, either good or bad. But I was disappointed, because I just wanted porn to look like real sex in the modern era. I wondered if this, the curated collection that now had made me sexually depressed, was as good as it was ever going to get.

A year later, the very store at which I'd purchased the catalog hired me as its porn reviewer. Say what? I saw that as my chance to right a wrong, at least for myself. I discovered the store's cache of adult video industry magazines and pored over their lurid, graphic pictures on my breaks. I was shocked by the pictures, yet turned on by the range of sexuality presented (albeit a narrow range). I felt excited by the women directors, disappointed by the female reviewers parroting the men around them, fired up by the ignorance about female pleasure, and appalled by the awful writing. Yet I was hooked. And while my employers included porn viewing in their mandatory sex education

training for employees, I felt it my duty as reviewer and consumer to go beyond the requirements for porn watching. Given
free rentals at the sex shop, I brought home as much porn as
would fit in my motorcycle bag. Over the months I saw a few
good films—some that really turned me on, many that didn't.

I was enjoying my job as a reviewer (in every sense), but that
didn't make being a female porn consumer any less confusing.
The feminists in my office were pro-porn, but anti–male sexuality. The porn industry was pro-itself, but ambivalent about
women enjoying sex—and clearly not supportive of nonformula
porn. The media in the outside world were unfailingly anti-porn,
unless they wanted ratings. Since the 1970s, conventional feminist thinking had rigorously informed the entire culture that
porn degrades women, so most people grew up thinking that
was true, without understanding what the statement even means
(or bothering to experience porn for themselves). As I read other
reviews while writing for the sex store, I noticed that, across the
board, all the writers took their stances on porn really seriously,
while never taking the consumer seriously at all. All these attitudes somehow managed to be visible in every porn video I watched,
whether it was an industry formula, Barbie-goes-through-the-
motions video, or a female-directed, no-male-ejaculation video.
I didn't fit in anywhere, yet there seemed to be a lot of women
like me. When we just wanted to jack off, all of this was enough
to make a girl lose her boner.

Amazingly, despite all this, I was finding good porn. Even
though I was watching porn every day, and you'd think I'd be
jaded, I saw porn that still made me hit "rewind" more than a
few times, and when I was at my computer surfing the Web
I started bookmarking hot sites. I was thrilled when (often

accidentally) I saw authentic female orgasms that had me grip-
ping my thighs together in stunned erotic empathy. I saw riveting
blow jobs that made my mouth water with envy. I found websites where pairs of women and men tore each other's clothes
off with passion that startled me. I watched films with gorgeous
cinematography, natural lighting, beautiful real people as performers. And I saw a whole host of independent porn that blew
my mind. Film noir porn, playful European porn, intelligently
staged voyeur porn that aroused and inspired me. I still couldn't
find any good bisexual porn, though, or porn that didn't see
male anal penetration as "gay" or "perverted," but I figured that
eventually high market demand would win out over mainstream
porn's puritanical perceptions of male and female sexual roles.
(I'm still waiting....) After all, with around 12,000 titles released
a year, I could always hope.

The Web changed everything for me, and for other female
porn consumers. It's changing porn even as I write this. I got
recognition on my own website writing about porn while I
worked at the women-run sex shop, but I still couldn't seem
to connect with anyone in the business who had ties to the outside world of consumers—namely, anyone who knew what
viewers really wanted. Working in the sex shop, I came to realize that porn's audience wasn't what everyone thought it was.
My porn reviews had gotten me much attention online, and the
salespeople in the store were thrilled that their reviewer was
making noise about women liking porn.

This was the reality every day in the retail stores and on the
mail order phone lines: we had oodles of female porn customers,
and they liked getting positive reinforcement about enjoying
porn. No one needed to be validated, but they warmly welcomed

a normal conversation about porn. Lots of women were enthusiastic about it, some even striding out with several porn titles
for a weekend. Every customer I chatted with about porn was
excited to have a real discussion about it, as if we were snark-
ing about the latest lame-but-entertaining Hollywood
blockbuster while discussing the merits (or not) of facial ejaculation or plot vs. all-sex videos, all while I rang them up for
lube and batteries. Making fun of so-and-so's scary new boob
job, like it was celebrity gossip. Talking about porn genres, like
one would compare action films to feel-good films. This was a
far cry from the image of lone male masturbators in raincoats.
Meanwhile, the rest of the porn industry (and media folk who
covered porn) pretended that I, my blog, my company, and others
like it simply didn't exist.

My porn review website was popular, enthusiastic email
rolled in from both women and men (even from couples writing together), and I got marriage proposals from 300-pound Elvis
impersonators. (I told them that Priscilla had left the building.)
People wanted more: more recommendations, more tips on finding good porn websites, more fun links to hot explicit photo
galleries, more resources for their porn libraries both online and
off. I made lots of friends in the fringes of the mainstream porn
business, and some friends who weren't on the fringes at all. I
was being interviewed by national cable news networks and
glossy magazines about my being a female porn reviewer and
about the attitudes of other females who consumed porn. I
blogged about porn until my iBook practically burned a hole in
my lap; and even though most of the porn movie industry is still
slow to "get" blogs and porn blogging, the online world of porn

blogging (and online forums) became the center of the porn resource universe for women and men alike, around the world.

I didn't stop there. I joined more online forums, posted questionnaires and polls, and accepted free rental memberships from friends working in porn stores all around San Francisco. I met hundreds—hundreds!—of women, thousands on one review site alone, who were interested in finding good porn. We traded tips, complained about things we hated, made fun of stuff that grossed us out, and helped each other find hot porn. Those many, extremely diverse women—what I named on an online forum, the Smart Girls' Porn Club—are the inspiration for this book.

Meanwhile, everyone who was making and selling porn felt at a loss for what a female audience might want. The mainstream adult industry seemed to think women only existed in couples, and that women's porn should be anemic, soft, dumbed-down with clearly contrived romance framing the same tired formulas. I was appalled that the porn industry was trying to dumb itself down more—was that even possible? There was simply no way I could explain the far-ranging (and I do mean far) voices and opinions of the women in online porn forums about the porn they preferred. They liked things that shocked me, they hated things each other loved, they were offended and aroused by some of the most extreme porn I've seen—sometimes, confusingly, having both reactions at the same time. The degradation question always came up and got discussed humorously and rationally; every girl saw it from a fresh (and sometimes surprising) angle.

All of this made me want to find good porn and share it with the club. The sad fact is that most women (and men) just don't know porn's best-kept secrets: anyone can enjoy it, and you have a choice—you don't have to watch bad porn. And you don't have to be a guy to like what you see.

Porn needs to be seen without sexual shame. Porn is a healthy way to experience sex, period. Women and men need to learn about fake female orgasms, and how to tell the difference. Porn, like Hollywood's reality TV, is often sexual disinformation: many sex acts are hot to watch but likely the sexual equivalent of *Jackass* and you shouldn't try them at home. Porn is awesome fantasy fodder, but it's also dumb fantasy usually made by people who rarely understand the sex acts they're portraying. Think about what you're looking at in context: degradation is in the eye of the beholder. Leave the homophobia at the door: porn (like most entertainment media) has homophobic tendencies and you need to evaluate male and female sexual roles for yourself. And even if you're color-blind, porn isn't: interracial videos fetishize skin color and often show fairly lame stereotypes of black people. It's more than annoying. So become a smart shopper, and vote with your credit card.

Mostly, porn should be fun, hot, wankable. But I think it can be pretty liberating, too. Set yourself up to challenge anti-porn pundits and sex-negative points of view by becoming a clever consumer armed with self-knowledge about porn's positive effects on your own sex life. If we're to really solve some problems, we need to break down cultural myths about porn's degradation of women, its mythical ability to cause rape and child molestation, and lies about how it creates "porn addicts." None of these myths can be borne out by unbiased, factual studies. The more smart girls there are who know the truth about what porn really can and can't do to each of us as individuals, the more that people who perpetuate these myths will lose a little power over our freedom of choice. And over our sexuality. So, welcome to the Smart Girls' Porn Club.

Violet Blue
San Francisco
March 2006

chapter 1

what a smart girl wants

Take a stroll to the grocery store, movie theater, or mall, and you'll have made contact with lots of women who watch porn. Seriously. Like the pod people in *Invasion of the Body Snatchers*, they can't be recognized just by looking at them—except maybe they've got a little more spring in their step. Women watching porn is still a taboo subject in our culture, but most women have caught a glimpse of porn, and a great many watch it regularly. The stereotype of a desperate man in a raincoat has faded like a B-movie special effect into our past. Today women, men, and couples of all orientations and of all walks of life participate in one of our favorite extracurricular activities: getting off to all kinds of porn.

Millions of average people a year in the United States rent, purchase, and enjoy pornography. Porn is watched not just by single men but by women, married men, and couples—with a diverse range of age, physical ability, sexual orientations, and backgrounds. Women-owned sex toy businesses that cater to female customers added explicit films to their stock about twenty years ago, and when they did they saw their businesses grow exponentially. Many of these women-owned sex shops see their porn sections as a reliably increasing area of revenue, and for these shops, single men are the shopping minority. Not to mention the growing number of porn websites created by women, for a female audience.

In the 1970s and '80s, pretty much the whole genre was being produced with men in mind, despite a number of notable exceptions. *Deep Throat* caused a stir of epic proportions in 1972, showcasing what was then an outrageous sex act (deep-throat fellatio), and even celebrities flocked to seedy movie houses to see it. In the same year, *Behind the Green Door* was shown to an enthusiastic audience at the Cannes Film Festival. As a result, women and heterosexual couples became visibly active consumers of porn. Through the 1990s women-owned sex shops were steady sellers of porn, and in the first years of the new millennium we witnessed an explosion of online female porn reviewers, shoppers, webmasters, directors, photographers, and moderators of porn forums. Not only were these businesses showing hot profits along with hot merchandise, but other adult retailers were also starting to realize that women were statistically increasing their market presence through purchasing power—and lots of straight and lesbian couples were watching porn, too. The mainstream porn industry responded by producing movies that it thought women might want to watch. The movies were mostly lame and stereotypical, but I'll get to that later.

The first time I watched an adult movie, I went on the recommendation of another smart girl who knew a lot about porn. She listened to my list of desires—good filming, great story line, and a dark edge—and recommended a video that totally disappointed me. Part of the problem was that her interpretation of what I described as a "dark edge" was a film full of overly macho porn dudes badly pretending to be gangsters—quite different from what I wanted to see; I had wanted something more fetish-y. But the main reason I stopped watching as soon as I'd started was that I expected a movie like the ones I was used to watching in theaters, not the cheaply filmed, overlit, poorly constructed video I ended up with. I expected a regular *movie*. And alas, the very Hollywood-looking and -acting actors in the movie turned me off, because they weren't anything like me or the people I could even imagine having sex with. The fake boobs, fake pearls, fake orgasms were more than I could bear.

Bringing myself to the point where I could comfortably select a DVD I'd really like and get off while watching it was a matter of my coming to know the unfamiliar, exciting, and arousing world of porn—a process of trial and error that involved watching many, many DVDs, both good and bad and everything in between. I came to view the process of trying out new porn movies as an ongoing sex experiment, one with which my lovers weren't always patient enough to help out. In my head I had an idea about the type of DVD and situations I most wanted to see depicted, and I allowed for that to change as I learned more about porn—and, at the same time, learned more about what turned me on. Now that I understand what I like, and how to find it, porn has become a sex toy that's as reliable to me as my trusty vibrator.

For newcomer and experienced porn viewer alike, porn can be a stocking stuffed with both candy and hand grenades. In this chapter, I offer a lot of suggestions that will help you define your fantasies and what you do—and don't—want to see in porn.

Be prepared to spend money renting or buying DVDs that don't work for you; it's the only way to find what does. Once you understand more about the porn world, you can be more specific when making your purchases or rentals or having pay-per-view online adventures, and you'll strike the jackpot more often than not.

Today women are proudly, loudly watching porn, and to my mind it's a happy sign of a much-needed change in women's sexual roles, especially as consumers. In our culture, women simply aren't exposed to as much explicit sexual imagery as men are, but this is all a-changing. One of the major obstacles that we women face in determining our own healthy vehicles for sexuality is the widely held notion that women don't respond to sexual imagery as men do—a notion that is absolutely untrue. In her 1994 study, Dr. Ellen Laan of the University of Amsterdam proved that women do, in fact, respond physiologically to sexual images. When seeing sex onscreen (whether from male or female directors), the women in the study responded, their genitals becoming congested with blood—a cornerstone of the sexual response.

Women Get Turned on by Explicit Imagery, Period

Guess what? The folks who said that women don't get turned on by explicit imagery were wrong. Like laughably antiquated notions about "female hysteria," getting turned on is *not* all in our heads, thank you very much. When we think about desire, erotic attraction, and arousal, we give all the credit to the functions of the higher brain—the thinking functions. We believe in our free will, our skills in making decisions to guide the more mysterious, more animalistic urges around sex. It has long been a hallmark of human nature that our sexuality is under volition; as rational people, we have no doubt that healthy sexuality requires self-control. Not a scrap of our sexual fantasies and desires (or so we think) is left completely on autopilot, just as even when we drive a car we consciously stay on the road. At least, until we see someone we're attracted to—and suddenly desire turns us right into monkeys, and we start acting like them.

Meaningful sexual motivation, it turns out, has little to do with physiological arousal. In fact, we get turned on by what we see, or by imagining or visualizing a sexual fantasy. Such visual creatures are we that our entire world is made up of images and feelings, together with the emotions and desires they trigger. At the same time, relationships are the bread and butter of who we are, with intimate relationships being a delicious main course for our psyches. Yet graphic erotic imagery sends a direct current buzzing from our brains to our groins. Face it: images turn us on, and they can get us off. That is, if we know how to use them .

Our desire for intimacy in relationships and our visceral response to porn may come from two different places in us, yet they aren't mutually exclusive. In our ideal relationships, the conscious act of desire and genital performance are not things we want separated; instead, we want the two working in tandem, like a perfect set of doubles in tennis. But porn is so immediate, so visceral, that it disrupts our rationality. We can't help but look at it, nor can many of us resist getting aroused by it. And because we want our seemingly mindless genitals to play nice with our relationships, the lack of control makes us feel like suddenly we're driving a car with no brakes. It's as if what's safe is always at odds with what's sexy. It doesn't have to be, but the act of bringing the two ideas together is a conscious one. It takes examining what porn really is, and how to use it.

Some people feel as intimidated by porn as they do by sex toys—though that's all porn is: a sex toy in a thousand different guises. It's an arousal tool to use with a partner, or alone. Looking at explicit imagery is still considered by some women to be something "dirty." But watching porn, in most cases, is simply a means to an end: the watcher's orgasm. End of story, and sleep tight. Watching porn can spice up a night at home with a lover, or be a solo masturbator's quick and reliable way to relieve sexual tension. People watch porn to get off on visual stimulation, because watching sex, sexy images, or fantasy scenarios makes us hot. And nothing gets to the point better than porn.

Why Does a Smart Girl Watch Porn?

In the quest to self-define our own healthy sexualities, let's pull back the curtain on all those average women who watch porn. What are all these smart girls *doing* with dirty movies? Why would any woman watch porn—and what can you get from it? The women who like porn have their own range of motivations. Most just want to get off seeing people have sex—it's that simple. Quite a few enjoy the notion that it's dirty to see anyone, especially women, being aggressive and acting sexually explicit, and the taboo titillates them.

Maybe the idea of watching two people get it on is on *your* top ten list of sexual fantasies. Whatever your attitude, porn is the safest way to explore voyeurism, period. Explicit sex onscreen seems to be a powerful aphrodisiac for lots of people—

and maybe it will be for you, too. It could be that you want to try out porn as a sex toy, the same way you might buy a new vibrator or play with a different brand of condom. Or the idea of doing something forbidden or naughty, or seeing a major taboo shattered, might be your flavor of the month. There are many reasons to watch porn, and you may find one, or several, of your motivations here.

Getting Off

The simplest, most basic reason to watch porn, of course, is "to get off." Many women use adult videos just as another person would use a vibrator—like a sex toy. Switch it on, it gets you aroused and pushes you over the top, then switch it off and put it away. You can masturbate to porn any way you like, anytime. It can be a fantastic sex toy that keeps you sexually healthy, in touch with your own arousal and orgasms, and visually in touch with what sex looks like (and sounds like). Porn can get you revved up before you go out, or it can be part of a hot date you have with yourself. Explicit visual stimulation has such a powerful arousal trigger—especially sex acts, scenes, or fantasy scenarios that fulfill a particular fantasy—that most women can use it reliably to bring themselves to orgasm.

Natural Curiosity

Aren't you wondering what the big deal is, anyway? Curiosity is a force to reckon with. Porn is everywhere: in the media, on TV specials, the topic of blockbuster movies. Porn stars are in mainstream magazines and have bestselling books, and you may have a friend or lover who has talked about watching adult videos—or bragged about dating a porn star. None of these things actually shows you any porn, or gives you an idea of what the movies, or their effects on you, are really like. Perhaps it's time to end the mystery.

Ever Seen Two People Have Sex for Real?

In California around the early 1980s, most of us who were kids in fourth grade were treated to a grand total of one hour of sex education. This consisted of the boys and girls being separated and shown animated films about reproductive anatomy, puberty's physiological changes, and the cycle of birth. It was great to learn where babies came from, but in terms of the whole of human sexuality and what we were going to discover as we became adults, these films in retrospect didn't seem related to sex at all. No one told us about pleasure, or what sex—or even actual, nonillustrated genitals—looked like. Many children in the United States didn't (and still don't) even get the one-hour lesson I received in school.

Porn can make up for this deficiency many of us share, and become part of your own personal erotic education. You might watch it to learn new techniques or moves, or to see how the pros do it. Although the people in porn usually don't look like "average" people—they're relatively skinny, augmented, made-up, and shaved or waxed—when they get down and dirty they show us what it looks like when people have sex. It's a wholly different type of sex education, and an essential one at that.

Unless you make love in front of a mirror or look at your (and your partner's) genitals up close, you may never have an accurate idea of what realistic genital topography is or what people actually look like when they're being sexually stimulated. For people who have concerns about how their genitals look, or feel discomfort with how their bodies appear to others, it's an eye-opener to see someone else's genitals eroticized—especially if they look like your own. And who *knew* there were so many variations in women's vulvas, all adding up to "normal"? I sure didn't, until I started watching porn. My sexual education grew by leaps and bounds as I watched porn, simply because I saw a variety of types of anatomy, and I truly got an education when I saw my first up-close female ejaculation: I saw how the muscles down there actually *moved* during a real female orgasm. While porn isn't great for learning about accurate sex techniques (since the film editing means that the whole of sexual activity isn't necessarily shown), it can—sometimes inadvertently—be an amazing learning tool, for a variety of reasons.

It's Fun for Couples
Glossy men's magazines like *Maxim* run plenty of articles that tell guys how to convince their gals to watch porn with them. What I wonder is, when will we see the article telling me how to get my boyfriends in line with the program? Watching porn with someone you're hot for, or want to get in their pants, is a real treat. So what's the allure, exactly? Easy—it's another sex toy that couples can share. The first time you try it with someone else, watching an explicit film is an experiment; either you'll think it's lame and turn it off, hopefully laughing, or you might feel a twinge of arousal...maybe more. And it can be fun for you both to watch hot sex, and to both be turned on at the same time. Porn is a versatile toy, too, because you can take turns watching, use your hands, imitate the people onscreen, or use the imagery to spark desire and move on to ignore the film altogether. How you use it together is up to you.

Couples who want to add a little spice to their sex lives can try out porn to turn up the heat. Conversely, they may watch a few films, find them anticlimactic (pardon the expression), and have hotter sex because they know they can do it better than the porn stars—and because porn *can* lack heat and chemistry between couples, it's sometimes true. But check your expectations: being merely a sex toy, porn only enhances what you've already got: it can't replace or "fix" anything.

New couples can add porn to an already-sizzling sex life to push their new sexuality to higher levels, or into new territory. Established couples, especially those with children or other time constraints, might enjoy having a very special adult "treat" that they can enjoy in their private time together. Those who find they like this versatile sex toy can add regular viewing to their sexual repertoire, perhaps mixed in with other variations like fantasy play and other, physical sex toys.

Find New Fantasies

In all honesty, most porn is pretty unimaginative. Like soap operas, it falls into basic formulas, and the scene endings are, well, predictable. But adult film is one of the only industries in the world actively, endlessly exploring and enacting human sexual fantasies, always on the lookout for new story lines, for new and exotic locations, for new ideas to depict on film, and even for new positions and sex acts to show the viewer. This makes it a unique place to look for fresh material for your own fantasy life, as it can spark ideas of things to try with a lover or a date. Often the scenarios might seem mundane, but you'll likely be surprised by the power of your libido when you become aroused seeing something from a fresh angle, or see a position you'd like to try, or even realize that you want to experiment with a new type of sex act, such as oral sex or S/M.

Tired of the same old image or stroke when you masturbate? You're not alone—the popularity of sex toys in general underscores the fact that most women enjoy variety in their masturbation. Porn is just another way of mixing it up.

See Things You'd Never Try Yourself
Sexual fantasies often aren't grounded in reality, or if they are, they're likely unrealistic in a big way—that's why they're *fantasies*. And that's okay; it's perfectly acceptable to fantasize about things you'd never actually try, never ask someone else to do to you. Sometimes you might find that these fantasies are beyond what you'd deem permissible for you to try in real life, and they might even seem disturbing. But know this: just because you fantasize about something doesn't mean you want it to come true. Fantasies of all stripes, from the benign to the extreme, can be found in porn, and this makes adult imagery an especially suitable arena to see something you'd never try yourself, but might enjoy masturbating to. This can range from fantasizing about same-sex erotic activities to getting off watching something you find potentially offensive—like facial come shots, gang bangs, or scenarios involving a hint (or a lot) of force. If it offends or really bothers you, then don't do it—but if you realize that you're simply watching consenting adults who seem to be enjoying themselves (and that it's just a job for them), and that watching them work doesn't change who you are in any way, you might feel free to use your forbidden fantasies to their full erotic potential.

Get What You Can't Find at Home

He won't go down on you? Watch it in porn! What if, over time, you realize that you'd like to try a different sexual activity with your lover, such as oral sex, and you ask her or him to try it, and your partner claims not to be interested? Well, you can drop the subject, never bring it up again, and mourn the loss of fulfilling a potential fantasy with your lover—though you may wind up frustrated and resentful over time. I don't recommend this route. You could also cheat on your partner, but that's almost always disappointing and ends badly. You could badger your partner, but that's no solution, either. You have a better choice: address your dilemma with little or no damage to your relationship, *and* find a satisfying way to enjoy your fantasy—by watching other people "do it" in porn. In addition, porn can be a great way to introduce a new erotic activity, such as oral or anal sex, into your life; if you watch a video together that has that sex act in it, it'll at least be easier to talk about afterward.

Our Fantasies Are About Fucking, Not Shopping

Are you as tired as I am of seeing popular media pushing stereotypes of women being more interested in shopping or money than sex? Or, worse, women using sex only as a tool for manipulation? Or glossy women's magazines that promise fifty sex tips, but always in exchange for "keeping" or "getting" a man, forever dancing around the explicit sex that might actually get us off? Porn consumption, by all estimates, is reaching an even split between male and female consumers; but still, magazines purportedly aimed at savvy sexual women won't even touch our porn-lovin' habits with a ten-inch...pole. Our fantasies are about more than that. Our sexual fantasies are important. And porn plays an important role in our fantasy lives—and vice versa.

Porn takes sexual fantasies (and fantasy sex acts) out of the realm of imagination and puts them up on the big screen, or the wide-screen TV, for all to see. Sexual fantasy is everyone's own private, personal sex toy. A good fantasy played out in your head can take you to dizzying heights of arousal, enhance an intensely private moment of masturbation, or illuminate an experience with a partner. Someone can have a scenario progressing in their head when receiving oral sex, act out their impulses with a companion, or tell their fantasies to a lover on the phone. But before we turn our fantasies into the unforgettable encounters we wish them to be, or prepare to see them onscreen, we first have to define what they are.

Sexual fantasy is the cornerstone of our individual sexual expression. An erotic fantasy is any thought, idea, image, or scenario that interests you sexually. It doesn't necessarily have to turn you on, though it can be the one thing that gets your blood boiling. And if you think you don't fantasize, think again. Fantasies can emerge from your erotic imagination in countless different forms, from fragmented to detailed. We may see famous people who are attractive and imagine that our lives intersect erotically. We can revisit memories of times we have enjoyed with earlier partners, using them to make us feel good in the present. Often, we envision scenarios that have never happened—and some that aren't even possible.

Sometimes we tell others what we've actually done, fantasized about, or want to do, making a fantasy for them—or us—come true. Whatever shape your fantasies take, exploring them can open doors to understanding your arousal, while at the same time enabling you to tap into new channels of erotic expression that work for you.

Some people don't care to explore their fantasies. Many others are more willing. Because those fantasies arise in our imagination, and therefore are connected with our subconscious, they can be startling, unpredictable, and sometimes even shocking. When we become aroused it's easy to surrender ourselves to whatever movie we're running in our heads, and play it faster in the direction that gets us closer to orgasm—but sometimes, afterward, we realize that what got us off went beyond what we think of as acceptable in our daily lives. It's easy to feel guilty after a fantasy has gone to a place or an act we find unpleasant or offensive. Admitting this guilt can make us feel shame about sex, our desires, even who we are. This is especially true when the fantasy was powerful and included something that in real life we would never do, like degrade ourselves or betray a loved one. When fantasies move toward the arenas of everyday life (as they're bound to do), they can manifest in ways that make us uncomfortable.

Sometimes it's not the content of the fantasies that can trigger guilt, but rather the time or place that they occur. Fantasies can happen at inconvenient times, such as at work or on the bus, creating a sexually charged situation in our heads while the world goes on around us. This may feel inappropriate or "dirty." Or fantasies can happen during sex with a partner: Your partner is fully present, yet unaware that you're imagining things, even acts with other people, to get yourself off. You might want to masturbate to a secret fantasy you see in an adult movie without your partner—or you might be witnessing your private fantasy while they're sitting right next to you. The illusion is created that somehow we've betrayed them. It's important to understand the role of sexual fantasy in sex before beating your-self up about what, how, when, or with whom you fantasize. We all know that fantasy is not reality. But when we mas-turbate and imagine troubling things, people, or situations, our human curiosity kicks in and we ask ourselves whether these things are what we really want. For some people this is a hor-rifying thought. It's important to keep in mind that fantasies don't necessarily bear any relationship to reality. The realm of fantasy is the sanctuary in your mind where you're free to enjoy things that you would never do in real life. And fantasy is not only the realm of the imagination where we can court the for-bidden, it's also a powerful sex toy that can be used to arouse, heighten pleasure, and attain orgasm.

Use Your Own Fantasies to Find Good Porn

Think about your fantasies for a moment, whether they're vivid, vague, seemingly mundane, or a little scary. Don't try to look deeply into their meanings, just pick out their main themes. What you're doing is isolating what makes them a peak erotic experience for you. Keep your mind open, and don't pass judg-ment on yourself—this isn't about being "good" and "bad," it's about coming to understand what turns you on. Note what stands out, and weigh the important differences between what's possible in fantasy and what's possible in reality. The fantasy types below can also help you make the right selections when looking for a porn film that will get you off.

- *Firsts:* first time with a sexual act such as penetration, oral sex, or anal sex

- *Loss of control:* someone wields sexual power over you, "makes" you do things
- *Having control:* exerting sexual power, having people "service" you on command
- *Taboo:* having sex with a forbidden person like clergy or family, an animal, same gender, significant age differences, inappropriate urges or timing, rape, nonconsent
- *Multiple partners:* a gang bang—one person with four or more partners, sex with the football team, threesome, sex party, orgy
- *Casual or anonymous partners:* strangers, the waitress, the UPS guy
- *Your current or past partner:* a memory of a real-life event; imagining a peak experience you hope to do together; imagining your partner behaving differently than usual, such as being dominant or submissive
- *Public spaces:* the office, movie theater, park, dressing room, your gym
- *Being "used":* a slave, a fuck toy, getting passed around
- *Role-play:* you or your partner is an icon: a cop, schoolgirl, hooker, doctor, teacher, human pony, dog owner
- *Gender play:* seeing women as men, men as women, or people who are both—that is, transsexuals
- *Romance:* dreamy settings—being seduced by a rock star or actor, making love tenderly to the girl at the office, getting rescued by a hot and horny fireman, saving your sexy fantasy lover from danger
- *Objectification/fetish:* breasts, butts, dicks, mouths, panties, shoes, leather

- *Voyeurism:* watching people have sex through the bushes or from outside their house, secretly seeing someone undress or masturbate, watching people have sex on TV, seeing other people—such as a single woman—view sex acts

Now you're getting an idea of your main fantasy components. Think about what your favorite themes are, or try on new ones that appeal to you. Feel comfortable with tapping into what these fantasies trigger when you want to become aroused. Remember that if you fantasize about something shocking, like being forced to perform sex, it doesn't mean that you really want it to happen or that you're a bad person. By identifying it in the realm of your fantasies, you can find a safe space where imagination fuels desire. By learning how to turn yourself on with fantasy, you can do extraordinary things, like make yourself hugely aroused and teach yourself a new masturbation technique. Or you can fantasize while your partner goes down on you, and learn to orgasm with the combination of their stimulation plus your fantasy. If you have a partner, and have established trust and good sexual communication, you can share your fantasies—you can even make some of them come true. And if you're looking for good porn showing some sizzling fantasies from your mental checklist, you'll have a better idea of what you want to avoid— or what you really want.

common concerns
about content

E veryone has concerns about porn. And many smart girls run up against these concerns when they want to watch porn— they are stopped, or their arousal is derailed by their concerns about content. Some women will put in a DVD, see something that offends or upsets them, hit the "eject" button, and never experiment with porn again. While it's true that everyone has concerns, and that there is probably something out there to offend everyone, most people don't know that their concerns can help them select the right video or website, and that the viewing choices in porn are many.

Porn Can't Make You "Do" Anything

If you're new to the world of porn, feeling afraid or unsure, or feel morally at question with an aspect of sex, it can bring up powerful feelings. Adding any new sexual behavior to your life can feel like a make-or-break situation, and sometimes it is. And porn touches on many issues that can be intense.

Much like old myths that masturbation will make you go blind or grow hair on your palms—myths once intended to scare people away from exploring what we now know is a healthy sexual practice—a few modern myths exist about people who watch porn:

People who watch porn are compulsive masturbators.
Masturbation is normal. Everyone masturbates, and people who watch porn have a range of masturbation practices, just like everyone else. We live in a culture that labels anyone who enjoys masturbation as "compulsive," despite the normalcy of this healthy human behavior.

People who watch adult videos are porn addicts who can't enjoy sex without onscreen stimulation.
It's quite true that some people can become habituated to certain stimuli (especially when they discover something that works well), such as a frequent erotic fantasy, a pet vibrator, or a favorite sexual position. When you find something that you really like (or that brings reliable enjoyment to sex), repeat use does *not* mean you are "addicted" to it—though if you'd like to change your masturbation habits or broaden your range, you can adopt new practices. Masturbation is the key method for incorporating new sexual practices, and by arousing yourself with masturbation by familiar methods, you can try new sexual behaviors while in your most familiar state of heightened arousal. Turn yourself on and try something new.

People who watch porn are child molesters.
Or:
Watching porn turns people into rapists and child molesters.
People who molest children are interested in children, not adult porn. Those interested in sexualizing underage kids will be much more interested in watching movies that feature young children than masturbating to images of explicit, adult sex. Adult porn is a voluntary arousal tool, like sexual fantasy (the imagination), erotic books, and sex toys, to name a few. They lack the power to "make" anyone do anything they do not already want to do.

Only people who can't have a "real" relationship watch porn.
This is one of the most hurtful myths, designed to shame people into sexual isolation. Retail statistics chart the skyrocketing sales and rentals of porn to couples, showing that couples as well as unpartnered individuals are using porn to enhance their relationships or to find release in between relationships. Some choose solitary pleasure, and porn provides a great release from sexual tension. Besides, taking time out to masturbate when you're in a relationship isn't cheating—it's taking care of yourself.

When you watch porn, you support a racist/sexist industry.
I partially agree on this one. Sexist stereotypes in porn? They're like wheat in Kansas. Racist stereotypes in porn? You bet. These issues have been huge struggles and pivotal turning points for many performers and directors, and thankfully, these directors and performers have turned many stereotypes on their heads, striking back and making their own hot, smart, porn—porn that even erotically comments on these stereotypes. To escape

the clichés, look for videos made by women, people of color, and independent production houses.

Porn makes viewers want more extreme sex or sexual material. That's like saying if someone tries hot sauce, they'll never be happy until they set their tongues on fire. Perhaps for some— but really, is *Edward Penishands* a gateway drug? Watching adult videos does not give you some unquenchable thirst to find something crazier, harder, more extreme—you already have this urge before you turn on the computer or TV. It's true that when you grow comfortable with porn you will crave variation—but always within the bounds of what's sexually comfortable for you.

How Do You Stack Up?

The number one fear or concern most women (and men) have about watching porn is that they won't stack up, or measure up, to the people they see onscreen. And whether they personally are comparing themselves to stars or starlets, or are worried that their lover might, they're right. After all, the people in porn look and act nothing like regular human beings.

Sure, they walk, they can talk (mostly), some can even snap their gum and have sex at the same time—and several have degrees in subjects such as entomology or microbiology and have very high IQs. But porn actors don't look (or have sex) anything like you or me, and that's why they got the job. Like Hollywood stars, porn stars are overblown caricatures of contemporary culture's ideals and inhabit a tiny end of the gene pool. The actors are all very limber, and can withstand extended periods of sex in difficult positions under hot lights.

They shave their balls, wax their asses, and sometimes wear makeup on virtually every inch of their bodies...and still perform. They can have sex with total strangers and make it look like it's not a job. It's *not* an easy job every day, but many actors make it look like pleasure.

Porn is fantasy, porn is fiction—even though the people up there having sex are flesh and blood. The films are heavily edited to make the sex last seemingly forever, to only show everyone's good angles, and to make the sex look like *way* more than it is. Everyone appears to be having a good day—no PMS, no stress, no wrinkles, no headaches, and definitely no flaws, fat, or disabilities. No one gets pregnant from unsafe sex, or gets an STD. Men are always turned on and stay hard forever. Women seem to magically have orgasms from the slightest stimulation! Bodies, true sexual response, sexual situations, and physical sex acts are not shown realistically in porn.

But still, we can't help but compare ourselves to the people we see onscreen. Porn can bring up a whole range of body-issues, from feelings of inadequacy over small breasts and penises, to worrying about your weight; from feeling ashamed of your vulva to wanting to hide the hair on your butt or back and the adult acne we all periodically fight. Porn, like Miss America contests, nudie magazines, television advertising, and music videos, can make us feel insecure about our desirability. It's also normal to worry that you or your lover might expect your sex lives to become like the sex you see onscreen, though this is unrealistic. Remember, porn actors are up there because they look different than everyone else and are willing to change their bodies (sometimes frightfully radically) to fit a fantasy "ideal." However, I think that precisely because it's so far away from reality, most of the industry's purported "ideal" that stars embody isn't what actually turns most of us on.

You might be worried that your lover will think porn stars are sexier than you are. Remember, porn isn't what we're supposed to be like. If you feel comfortable enough, tell your partner that you're worried about fitting into a fantasy ideal. You can always do some nonjudgmental poking around and ask your partner why he or she wants to watch porn, and then hear your partner out. Chances are good you'll hear it's because it turns your partner on, or might turn *you* on—not because they prefer blondes. Let your partner know that you want to stay your lover's number one fantasy fuck.

It's Offensive but It Turns Me On

Comparisons, judgments, and fear of the unfamiliar aside, you might have other worries. You might worry about seeing something offensive or disgusting that will be a turnoff—or worse. The chances of this are high in a film genre with the sole purpose of showing, in as much detail as possible, the vivid and explicit act of sex—a topic that is already difficult for some women to explore. Remember to include the judicious use of the remote control in your viewing habits. And try to inject a very necessary sense of humor about porn into your porn watching. This is, after all, the film genre that brings you such titles as *Bat Dude and Throbbin, Shaving Ryan's Privates,* and *Terrors from the Clit.*

It's unsettling to feel aroused by images we find offensive on one level or another. If you're ashamed of sex, you're likely to feel embarrassed by the explicit imagery in porn. Sexual surprise, offense, and shock manifest in several guises: embarrassment, shame, anger, depression, self-hatred—and confusingly, arousal.

If you find the image of another woman being graphically penetrated upsetting, yet simultaneously arousing, you will likely feel alarmed by your own feelings. But for most women, watching other women have sex is incredibly arousing, not upsetting or degrading. Some experience the seemingly contradictory feelings of upset and arousal, and find that it enhances their experience. Those comfortable with their sexuality and personal boundaries may enjoy visiting the experience of upset/arousal much like a roller coaster ride, or a scary movie. The best way to understand your reaction to porn, female sexuality, and your own sexuality is to examine your feelings. Are you ashamed of your own body, fantasies, or desires? Think about what you really want: hot sex in a healthy relationship, comfort about your own sexuality, or making your sex life more fun and adventurous. Make your goal a great sex life—in whatever definition you prefer and whatever style you feel comfortable—instead of feeling bad or worried.

Porn is in the eye of the beholder. It's degrading to you if you're degraded by it. Situations where people are behaving offensively onscreen can make anyone feel pretty bad, but on a personal level, you can call the shots about who or what makes you more (or less) of a person. And don't forget: unless you talk to the people who worked in the video that upset you, you'll never know how they felt about the experience.

But what if you have no problem watching graphic sex, but the content of what turns you on is something you find morally offensive, like a gang-bang, "forced" sex, or taboo fantasy situations? Getting off on a fantasy of female degradation can be extremely confusing, especially if you align your personality with strong beliefs about female power. It could be that these kind of fantasies allow your sexual id just the release it needs, much like the powerful businessmen who frequent dominatrixes for role-reversal (and no, it's no myth). Or, maybe it's the shock and surprise that arouse you; the stereotypes of the powerful male and the submissive female; the lack of control in the fantasy; the violent male desire for the woman; the sheer "wrongness" of it all; or the BDSM overtones in the filmed (and legal, work-conscripted) exchange that is part of the porn video. No matter what aspect of the offensive fantasy gets you going, ultimately it's a fantasy and the people in the video, on the website or in the pictures are performing, have signed legal releases, and are working to convey the fantasy (or in some cases, part or all of the fantasy/fetish has been faked). And just because you fantasize about something never, ever means you want it to happen in real life, nor does it make you a bad woman.

Does Porn Degrade Women?

For most people, the idea of a woman being degraded, shamed, or violated for someone else's viewing pleasure just isn't arousing. A number of people have strong convictions about pornography and women; some of these folks believe that graphic erotic images of women are harmful, from paintings to QuickTime videos, regardless of either the participation level of the woman in the image or the intent of the viewer. Another perspective sees porn as an industry that forces women into humiliation and sexual slavery. After all, no woman in her right mind would do something like that. Not for pleasure. Or would she?

Those who believe in porn's alleged degradation of women are making a lot of assumptions about the people in porn, specifically the women, and about the people viewing the imagery:

- The woman is ashamed of what she is doing—or should be.
- She isn't enjoying it, or women as a class can't and don't enjoy certain types of sex.
- She is sexually receptive and therefore less than human.
- The viewer is always male.
- The actress doesn't know the effect her image has—that porn leads to real-life acts of rape, child abuse, and degradation.
- Open sexual desire is shameful for all participants, on- and off-screen.

How can anyone possibly know how every viewer or participant feels, or sees him or herself as? The answer is that no one can. Each individual must be allowed to decide what is healthy and okay for him or her—no one else can decide that for you, or for another person.

Fake Breasts Freak Me Out

This is a big complaint among both female and male viewers. And porn *is* a heavily augmented industry, right up there with professional dancing and modeling and Hollywood acting. The business of the body, the image, requires focus on the performer as product, and many women (and men) mold themselves to standards of conformity or what they read as popular desire in their quest for success—and in both Hollywood and porn, surgical augmentation has been the norm. In Hollywood as in the porn industry, the average for augmentation procedures, such as liposuction, is every six months.

I'll argue that physical beauty is very much in the eye of the beholder—what's hot for you is a turn-off for someone else. Some women who watch explicit films get turned on by large-breasted women, and our mass culture feeds the stereotyping of big breasts equaling sexiness. Adult actresses and strippers find across the board that when they get their boobs done, lo and behold, they make more money. The problem is that you can usually tell when those breasts are fake, and a lot of women (and men) find them, well, kinda creepy. You can often see incision scars around the nipples, under the breast, adjacent to the armpit, or on the side. Implants make the breasts sit up quite high and move in a way that looks very different from natural breasts (if they move much at all). When the actress leans over they often look lumpy. And the very presence of evident implants can remind the viewer of surgery—not very arousing.

Not all porn actresses have surgery, though, and there are lots of hot all-natural gals out there. But some get a series of surgeries, and a few have unusual procedures performed. Some porn actresses have had cosmetic surgery on their labia and clitoris to make their genitals look more lean, and I know of at least one actress who had cheek implants so that her face would look more sculpted when she gave blow jobs. Breast augmentation became very popular in porn in the late 1980s, turned into an adult industry standard in the 1990s, and is now becoming less of a standard as the adult industry finds its market expanding to a more opinionated, more critical viewership.

It's not easy, but you can narrow down your viewing choices to watching films that feature all-natural women. There's more porn for this preference appearing on the market every day. Entire series cater to viewers who prefer natural women, and some big-breasted series even employ only naturally endowed women. Certain films and series don't market the women as "all-naturals" but will use them exclusively anyway. And you can almost always find all-natural women in independent porn and instructional videos. Use the "fast forward" button judiciously to find the actresses who turn you on for whatever reason, and don't be shy about acknowledging those reasons. Also, learn the names of stars whose physical endowments—surgically enhanced or not—turn you on, and avoid the ones you don't want to see.

I Don't Like Anal Sex/Oral Sex/Lesbian Scenes/ Facial Come Shots...

It's difficult to avoid these popular sex acts in porn. While anal sex with women as the recipient was rarely seen in the hetero-sexual films of the 1970s and 1980s, by the 1990s it had become a standard. A few videos here and there have no anal, and very few of director Candida Royalle's films have anal sex in them. But usually anal, oral, and girl–girl scenes are part and parcel of the porn formula, so get your "fast-forward" finger in shape.

The Men Only Come on the Outside of the Women, and the Women Never Come At All

No, it's not a typical sex practice anywhere outside porn, but external ejaculation is another of porn's standard practices, one nearly impossible to avoid. The practice of men pulling out to come has been around as long as porn. This is done so that the audience can see the orgasm, the peak and release of the sex act. It's the proof the guy came. Until recently, from the medical community to the adult community, little value was placed on female orgasm, and so male orgasm was—and still is—the centerpiece. Most viewers love to see a woman really getting off, but the makers of porn have been slow to focus on authentic female orgasms—or to even figure out what they are and how to make them happen. More and more films are coming out that focus on female pleasure, and on the women getting off, for real.

Only in the past twenty years have shots of facial ejaculation, or "facials," become commonplace in porn. Some women (and men) find this degrading or disgusting, while others—including many female viewers—find it highly arousing. Still others couldn't care less where the guy comes as long as they can see it. Some people think facials are boring and predictable, and would rather see the come shot on another body part they prefer. If you dislike facials, look for porn from independent filmmakers.

How Do They Do It with Those Fingernails?

Good question. Many female porn stars have fingernails that look like talons from a vicious bird of prey, and quite a few women see the stars fingering themselves on screen and wince. Those fingernails look like they'd be difficult to rub a clit with—and they definitely don't look safe for insertion. As with everything in porn, use the "fast forward" button without hesitation if fake nails bother you, but also know that those porn star nails are not the stick-on kind. They're acrylic, made part of the actual fingernail, and can't come off to stay lodged in any body cavity.

And usually they're not as sharp as they look but quite rounded at the tips. Also, these women are pros, and have had a lot of practice not scratching themselves or their partners.

The Genital Close-ups Are More Medical Than Sexual

Close-ups are the industry standard. With the exception of independent adult films and porn directed by certain women, you're going to be watching giant, floating, seemingly dismembered and brightly lit penises going into overlarge, surrealist vaginas, mouths, and asses on your screen. No mystery, no question about what's going on here—and that's part of the reason you'll see it. It might feel more like a documentary than a sexy movie, but these shots are the bread and butter of porn. The close-ups present the sex right there, in your face, without the distraction of the actors to take your attention away from one thing—the onscreen sex and its direct relationship to your masturbation. While close-ups are a little much for some people, seeing sexual anatomy in motion is an expectation that many viewers have when watching a video for masturbation purposes. Still, I'll agree that it's boring when that's all you get, with nothing else to tweak the imagination. If you don't want to see any close-ups, you can watch soft-core versions or films from selected indy filmmakers.

The Unsafe Sex Really Upsets Me

In porn's intent to portray harmless fantasy, it often gives us a fantasy world that can only ever be that: pure fantasy. While on a good day porn delivers the fantasies well, in the realm of portraying healthy and safer sex it will always fail. The main reason is that mainstream pornographers want to give viewers the fantasy sex they demand, and this version of sex doesn't require condoms, doesn't allow for the possibility that hepatitis can be transmitted by toys that have been inserted anally, and doesn't worry its pretty little head about the many dangers of unprotected sex with multiple partners or strangers. Instead, we get our fantasies, *and* a huge misrepresentation of how to stay alive and actively sexual in today's world. And no, it's not realistic at all, and porn is *never* a teaching tool in this aspect. If you're old enough to be watching porn, then you know better about safer sex.

True, a significant number of porn stars have been diagnosed with STIs—including a few cases of HIV/AIDS—while working in the business (and "working in the business" means having sex with other actors). The most famous case was legendary überdick John Holmes, who made films and had unprotected sex with actresses on-camera after testing positive for HIV in the 1980s. Holmes did not inform his coworkers, and put many people's lives at risk. In the late 1990s, Marc Wallice contracted HIV and continued working, infecting four of his female costars. Call it ignorant or call it murderous, their actions sent a wake-up call to everyone who works in porn. HIV isn't the only thing you can get from unprotected sex. Herpes, syphilis, genital warts, gonorrhea, chlamydia, bacterial infections, and other diseases and viruses can be passed by one single encounter sans condom.

Former adult actress Sharon Mitchell saw the risks far outweighing the benefits of working in adult films, and responded by founding AIM, the Adult Industry Medical Healthcare Foundation. In 1998 the adult entertainment industry suffered an HIV outbreak involving many people that Mitchell knew when she was in movies. The industry gave her the support that she needed to found AIM, a nonprofit organization serving sex workers and the general public in areas of HIV testing, STD testing, GYN services and treatment, counseling of many types, and sponsoring industry-related educational groups as resources for informational materials. Since its inception, AIM has successfully lowered the spread of HIV in porn, and has certainly increased awareness among performers. By adult industry standards, an adult entertainment worker should be tested for HIV/AIDS every thirty days, and though much of the industry supports mandatory monthly testing for chlamydia and gonorrhea, there is no standard for testing for other STDs. Most—though not all—producers/directors will not hire an actor if he or she lacks an HIV test less than 30 days old, while testing for other STDs is on a case-by-case basis depending on performers and directors.

Questions of Age and Consent: Bangbus and Paris Hilton

The women in porn participate on every level, from actresses who do it proudly for the money and those who have their hottest, most orgasmic sex while being filmed (and lecture at colleges about their articulate point of view), to actresses who do something they feel bad about, but do it nevertheless. However, the women who feel bad about it are in the minority and don't stick around long. It's just like every other job—some have a passion for the work, others see it as an enjoyable moneymaking activity, while some have mixed feelings about how they're making a buck, and for still others porn is just a job. Some women can get off on living out their sexual fantasies: letting themselves be watched, being the center of affection and attention, getting sexual with other women, getting sexual with a stranger, trying new fantasies in erotic role-play scenarios, and, yes, acting out being used or degraded. Make no mistake, there is never a point when the actresses are not doing what they want to be doing; they can walk off the set at any time. To get a fresh perspective on this, explore the writings (and films) from women who have enriched their sexual, political, and spiritual lives working in adult films, such as Nina Hartley's *Guide to Total Sex*, *How to Make Love Like a Porn Star* by Jenna Jameson, *Naked Ambition: Women Pornographers and How They Are Changing the Porn Industry* by Carly Milne, Annie Sprinkle's *Post Porn Modernist*, and Carol Queen's *Real Live Nude Girl: Chronicles of Sex-Positive Culture*.

A lot of women want to be in porn. It's lucrative, it's exciting—but it's also hard work and a tough field to be successful in. To be cast in porn, the performers have to want to be (and must prove that they will be) a reliable and interesting performer—otherwise, pornographers will pass them by, moving on to the next exciting new prospective talent. But once a performer finds a director or producer who says "okay, you're hired," the performer must provide a valid ID (with the performer's real name and age), any other names she or he has performed under, and sign a release: all according to 2257 federal law. The ID and information are collected prior to the shoot, copies are made, and then they are kept on file at a physical location that is given on both the box cover of the film as well as in the credits of the film itself. The address is clearly visible, with the time, title, and date of production.

The same goes for every video, from the low-rent to the latest "leaked" celebrity sex tape: if you're reading or hearing about it, that means every single person in the film has signed a release, completed the necessary 2257 requirements, and anyone promoting the video has access to all of the legal 2257 documentation, or where it can be physically located if asked. There is no such thing as a "leaked" or surprise sex tape; not unless someone wants to get sued, go to federal prison, or both. A website like the reality porn pioneer Bangbus bases its sexual interactions around a group of guys picking up girls "off the street" and convincing or "making" them perform sex on camera in a bus, making it seem like a surprise, as if they hadn't pre-screened the women and had all the documentation taken care of beforehand. The number of questions I get about the authenticity of these videos attests to their believability; they're poorly filmed, it's got a "reality" feel to it, and it's not hard to fake the whole scenario, but in reality, it's all contrived. My favorite versions of these are the gay series' where they "convince" straight boys to "try out" gay sex in a moving vehicle or other falsely spontaneous setting—a hot fantasy, for sure.

Who Are the Women in Porn?

All kinds of women are attracted to working in porn; they come from all walks of life, and in all shapes and sizes. Porn performers are selected for their gigs based on appearance, willingness to perform, and physical skills. They keep their jobs and become successful if they are reliable and relatively easy to work with, have a "glow" or magnetism, are above average in conventional standards of attractiveness, or can act (though not always a requirement), and they shine with a certain lust for sex. Porn folks, like their Hollywood counterparts, are very regular-looking people, just packaged very, very well with lots of makeup, professional hair styling, body waxing, lighting (and airbrushing for photos), and many having had some type of surgical augmentation.

The porn industry has filmed thousands of male and literally tens of thousands of female performers. Many will work for a few years, and then switch occupations, which makes keeping track of them difficult. Some get out to make better money elsewhere, because they find the work distasteful, or because it's tough to hack it in an industry that is hard on your body and psyche and is irritatingly obsessed with youth. But those who do stick around are star-quality, and amazing to watch at work. Newcomers are thrilling, and experienced players emit a focused heat onscreen.

Most women in porn start out as strippers or erotic dancers in clubs. Several will work a nationwide circuit of clubs, and make the move to porn slowly, or all at once if their first few films are successful. The really lucky women will rise to the top, winning awards for performances, becoming "contract girls," or grabbing the reins and writing and directing their own porn. Most women in porn also work the nationwide strip circuit for their entire careers as a lucrative adjunct to their film work.

Contract girls are women who are such hot tickets that a big production company, such as VCA or Vivid, will sign them to exclusive contracts. These women are respected and well paid, and though they can only work for one company they have a lot more say in the projects they're involved in than other performers. Often, outside of major companies, the women and men have no say in whom they work with or what project they're working on—it's a job like any other.

But what kind of women make porn? All kinds, for a variety of reasons, and from all walks of life. The mythology of the girl with "no where else to turn" heading into a life of porn because it's the lowest form of employment a woman could have is quickly fading into a legend of the past. A porn star like Jenna Jameson has written a *New York Times* bestseller, is the CEO of her own multimillion dollar company, and has fame equivalent to many Hollywood A-listers; this is clearly a sign of the times for what it means to be a woman in porn. Being a female porn star is now highly competitive, lucrative, and getting to the top means being business savvy and building an empire—and it's especially important to note that Jameson has always only ever done sex acts and scenes she prefers, rather than the popular conceptions that women in porn do things against their will or better judgment.

In fact, it's just the opposite: women in porn chart their own career choices, and consent of the female performer is the name of the game. It's easy to believe the hype about "leaked" celebrity sex tapes, such as the infamous Paris Hilton porn video, but don't be fooled. You better believe that distributor Red Light District had Paris's (and her lover's) 2257 permissions in place before the video was available in any shape or form. Think anyone's lawyers wouldn't love to take down a porn company? So-called "leaked" celebrity sex tapes have nothing to do with exploitation, and everything to do with publicity and vanity.

Celebrities and celebrity porn stars aside, most of the women in porn are there to make some money. Some women enter the business with a pro-sex, feminist agenda (like Nina Hartley,

Joanna Angel, April Flores, and many more), while others have no agenda except to make some cash. Like any other business that trades on looks and being in front of a camera, porn performers' self-image ranges from high to low, and everything in between. Some women actively want to change porn from within; others just want to pass through and get their bills paid.

But the question is, do the women having sex onscreen like what they do? Yes, no, and maybe. Some say they do, some avoid the question, and some repeat whatever they think their audience wants to hear: the real answer is in their character and presence onscreen. In the following chapters, I'll explain how to find videos and performers having authentically hot, enjoyable sex, and how to avoid performers and videos where actors just "go through the motions."

chapter 3

i was a porn virgin

A side from mouse clicks or pro-porn boyfriends, the context for your first foray into porn may not intentionally be a sexual one, solo or otherwise. You might watch your first porn film when your best friend drags you to a bachelorette party, or when a pal suggests something wild, like renting a dirty movie. If you decide you're okay with going along for the ride, know that you're doing just that—it's likely that your friend or friends were too nervous to watch porn on their own, and wanted to have you there to make it feel safer. It can be a lot of fun to watch porn with friends, and with the right crowd you might wind up laughing your head off. Prepare yourself by knowing that there's a chance you might see something that will arouse you or offend you, and realizing that, you'll be better able to disengage from seeing explicitly sexual material with people you don't feel sexual about. However, if you'd like to consider adding porn to your erotic repertoire, I recommend that you watch your first porn by yourself.

Women who watch porn alone and solely for themselves know what they like, enjoy trying new things, feel confident in making their own sexual choices, and like to treat themselves to masturbation on their own time and on their own terms. This reality is light years away from the decades-old, false stereotype of porn viewers as male, raincoat-clad, drooling, compulsive masturbators. Whether done by a gal enjoying time with her roommates gone, the mom with a quiet evening to spare, a girl whose boyfriend is out of town for the weekend, or just as part of a healthy masturbation session, watching porn ignites routine masturbation with a visceral erotic spark.

When you explore porn, you should do so without anyone else around to make you feel self-conscious, nervous, or worried about how you're feeling or reacting to what you see. That includes your lover, your best pal, the hottie you want to seduce, and anyone who might interrupt you with an uncomfortable surprise. Make sure your housemates are really not coming home, the kids are away, your sweetie is at work—check off all important items on your mental list so that you'll have total solitude and privacy.

When you're ready, make sure you have everything you need and will be undisturbed. If you can, eliminate possible distractions. Nothing is worse than taking your erotic temperature by watching a little porn, getting turned on, and experimenting— and then having the phone ring, bringing your arousal crashing down to earth. Unplug or turn off your phone, and don't try to multitask with any chores. Focus on the imagery. You may or may not like it or even get turned on, but you'll want to be able to assess for yourself how you feel. If you're worried about privacy and sound, make a mental list of what will make you feel safe; close your doors and windows, and keep the volume at a comfortably low level (or use our iPod).

Tips for Solo Viewing

Learn your own sexual anatomy before playing with porn. Read the anatomy chapter in your favorite sex guide, sit down naked with a mirror, explore your genitals with your hands.

Set aside some time for yourself when you'll be free of obligations and have some privacy.

Treat yourself to something sensual first, like a relaxing bath, a lush body lotion, or an aphrodisiac taste-treat.

Grab the remote, a towel, lube, a vibrator, a dildo or other sex toy, something to drink, and a just-in-case cover-up like a blanket.

Hit the "play" button. At first, pay more attention to yourself than the DVD. Using lubricant, caress your genitals, lingering in the spots that feel best. Take note of your favorite spots.

Tease yourself. When something feels really good—as in imminent-orgasm good—back off and touch yourself somewhere else, such as your nipples. This prolongs your pleasure and can make your orgasm really intense.

Try watching porn in different positions. You can sit in a chair, lie on your belly or back, or experiment with legs open or closed.

If you'd like to learn a different technique for masturbation or orgasm, get yourself aroused—*very* aroused—by watching a scene that gets you hot while using your regular masturbation technique. Slowly introduce the new behavior, such as trying anal penetration. You can also use this arousal technique to try things that may be ordinarily challenging, like deep throating a dildo. You can also experiment with prolonging orgasm.

Indulge yourself! Let your fantasies run wild. Become anyone, including the people onscreen. Orgasm as many times as you can— or come quickly, and hard. Be as nasty or as sweet as you like, and relish spending some truly decadent time giving yourself much-earned pleasure. Forget about the rest of the day; this time is for *you*. You're taking time out to take care of yourself and your body, and to make yourself feel good—something we never do enough. You deserve it!

Now set the scene for your porn adventure. You can look at porn on the sly, when no one's around, or you can make it a hot date with yourself. You can even get yourself in the mood by masturbating a little before the video starts.

Two Viewing Requirements:
Your Libido and Your Remote

Since porn is more of a sex toy than a "sex aid," it will add to (not fix) the current state of your libido. So, just as with any other sex toy, it helps if you're aroused before you begin watching porn. When you're ready to put the tape in and press "play," be sure to have the following items ready: lube, dildo, vibrator, towel, or all of the above, plus the remote control. Having a sex toy ready if you need it is handy; if the video turns you on and you want to get off, you won't have to interrupt your pleasure to search around for your toys.

But why the remote control? It's the only really required item for porn viewing: you'll need to fast forward through anything you don't like, or whatever distracts you from your arousal—be it lame dialogue, a sex act you don't care for, or a performer who leaves you cold. For some people this may seem like a hassle at first—why, you ask, can't the industry just make good porn?

The makers of porn try to appeal to as many tastes as possible in a relatively short amount of production time; they're also controlled by distributors who have fairly antiquated ideas about sex and sexuality—and especially about what people really want to see. Also, porn has to get to the point pretty quickly to retain horny viewers who usually want instant gratification, and so, as in Hollywood, the folks who make porn have boiled down their scenarios into formulas based on what they think viewers want.

Your First Shopping Trip

Before you make your first purchase or rental, make a fact-finding mission to the store or online retailer, so that you don't become overwhelmed by all the assaulting DVD covers with their explicit photos, attention-grabbing titles, and utter lack of order. Check it out, and plan to make a purchase on your second time around. On your maiden voyage, have a checklist in your mind of what you want—specific movie titles, actors, directors, series, or sex acts. Making an actual list is very helpful. Don't get your heart (or other parts) set on one video only, in case they don't have it or it's checked out—be prepared to be versatile.

When visiting stores in person, it takes a conscious effort to enter the porn section for the first time, and as a woman be prepared that most men who were browsing before you came in will flee. I kind of like it—I get the section to myself. But just ignore everyone else, and help yourself to what's rightfully yours as an adult. If you decide to go to an adults-only store where you'll have a better selection, men may not flee, but you might be the only woman in sight, and it can feel...conspicuous. Then again, you could be surprised to see other women and couples shopping for porn and sex toys: it's happening more and more every year.

If your town has one of the nation's many warm, welcoming, women-friendly sex toy stores, don't hesitate to shop there for your porn with the aid of the knowledgeable staff that run the registers. The workers in these stores typically know a bit

about the porn they carry and can point you in the right direction. Your first experience in one of these "clean, well-lighted"
places to shop for sex toys will be a shock—no sleaze! Many
of these stores are designed and run like upscale boutiques, but
without the cheesy element of "novelty" adult stores. As a customer, you'll be joining the (literally) millions of other women
and men shopping in these stores—people of every stripe and
persuasion, having fun renting and buying porn, and also purchasing vibrators, cock rings, and other sex toys. Unfortunately,
these terrific shops are found only in a few major cities (see chapter 9, Porn Resources for Smart Girls).

Most major cities have a selection of adult toy, book, and
video shops that are somewhat (or even very) sleazy and uncomfortable to shop in, generally because they aren't clean or kept
up in any visible way, and the clerks and even the customers
don't seem to want to be there. However, not all adult shops
are like this, and some will have female staff, witty gay clerks,
or an owner who works behind the counter and has a wealth
of knowledge to share—even if it's just knowing on which shelf
to find a particular title. Many adult shops have an arcade in
the back, where men pay to test drive the videos. This is a little
unsettling for those who aren't familiar with this culture, and
many women might feel worried about going into a store with
an arcade; keep in mind that arcades have been around since
the invention of moving pictures, reaching a heyday in the 1950s.
Unsettled to know that men are masturbating in the back while
you shop? It happens every day and night, even holidays. Smart
girls call 'em "jack shacks." See—now they're just funny.

The best way to handle nervousness is to march right in during
daylight hours, bringing a friend or two and ignoring everyone

else. But believe me, after years of going into every kind of porn store imaginable to do research, I'll bet cash money that if you're a woman and you go into one of the seedier shops, you'll be the only one in the store within two minutes. Our culture is so packed with sexual shame that whenever I walk into a jack shack to find a DVD, the men run for cover, leaving me free to take my sweet time shopping for my next rental.

Your local mom-and-pop video stores will have a closed back room where they keep the adult DVDs, away from the tender eyes of those under eighteen. Some stores opt to save on space and will have their video selection in large books that are kept behind the counter, containing box covers in a sort of big flip-book. If you don't see an annex for the porn, or a room with western-style swinging doors, ask to see the porn books. Expect that the adult titles will be more expensive than what you usually pay for a rental—they are much less likely to be returned than other videos, and retailers like to have insurance against losing their stock (hence the higher prices).

You might wind up going to more than one store to find what you want or a place where you feel comfortable shopping. You don't have to settle for the first place, or the nearest store, if you don't like it—remember, *you're the customer*. If you look around, you'll find what you're looking for, and if you have a particular title in mind you can always call ahead to see if they have it; some stores will set titles aside for regular customers.

Privacy and discretion are two main concerns for in-person (offline) porn shoppers. You can choose to peruse stores away from your home and work. Or go rent your videos when the store isn't busy, like on a weekday. You can have your lover rent for you—make it an erotic command if you like. Or you can just not give a damn what anyone thinks about your private sex life. And don't concern yourself with what the person behind the counter thinks about you, unless they're being inappropriate, of course. They've seen it all before, and they're probably worrying about theft, getting their Friday night shift covered, register balances, or the various problems porn store clerks contend with.

Many women choose to buy and rent their porn through the Internet. If discretion is an issue for you, then the Internet is your friend. The privacy that the Internet affords has made it both easy and safe for everyone to try out new sexual ideas and explore new possibilities, plus it puts porn within our reach. The Internet's drawback is that ordering and renting videos can be dicey if you don't know the company's privacy policy (some companies sell your information to other parties), and you can't ask anyone questions about the porn. That is why porn DVD review sites like Adult DVD Talk are invaluable.

Renting or purchasing online is an easy, private, and simple way to find and obtain the porn you're looking for. Some people find it a big pain to deal with the organizational chaos of finding stores and wasting travel time (including parking, in big cities) merely to rent porn in person, and are overjoyed to find that online transactions have quieted these complaints. Purchasing online is as simple as buying a book, and renting is just as painless, though each online store has its own policies and rules about rentals.

Rental sites are usually the best resources for finding and selecting what you want. They typically have excellent search engines, allowing you to search by title, director, actor, or genre (such as lesbian, heterosexual, or bisexual), and sometimes by studio, such as VCA or Evil Angel. They cater to a smorgasbord of tastes and sexual orientations, and might have suggestions that help turn up tasty selections for you. Then, you make your choice by clicking the "rent" button, at which time the site will drop that item into your virtual shopping cart and allow you to shop for another video. Online renters usually limit how many DVDs you can select—up to three is standard, but some go up to eight—plus a time limit for how long you can hold onto them. Most sites will let you hold your selection video while you shop for up to an hour, but then return the video to the "shelves" so others can shop for it, too. When ready to check out, you set up an account with a required credit card, and pay for your rentals. Each company has a different rental pricing structure; some are per rental, while others have a flat monthly fee. The rentals are shipped to you in discreetly marked packages—these businesses want your return patronage!—and you keep the videos for a set number of days, usually a full week. The rentals arrive typically within a few business days, and include a return envelope with postage. You watch the DVDs as many times as you like, then drop them in the mail when you're done.

Keep Your Expectations in Check

In mainstream low-budget porn, which comprises the major-ity of what's available through local retailers, online streaming video/clip websites, and DVD rental sites, the quality you're going to see is roughly that of regular (nonerotic) independent films, daytime soap operas, or daytime made-for-TV movies. These films feature simple sets, usually indoor filming in one location, standard harsh lighting, digital cameras (which are what contribute to their daytime TV look and feel), and barely present acting. Big studio films, by contrast, can be surprisingly complex in script, have terrific cinematography, and show sexy, believable actors, though the movies (and actors) have a purposely packaged and polished finish. Not surprisingly, the biggest studios have bigger budgets, access to better sets, actors who might have gone to acting school, writers with writing experience, and directors who are more likely to take their craft seriously. Some even use real film stock in their movies, which is costly but produces a higher-quality film, in look and feel. Sound quality, however, is generally poor, even in the big-budget feature films. The independents can have the same quality range, but they're less likely to be found in a neighborhood video rental shop; they can be found more easily online or in a sex toy or lingerie boutique.

Not all porn has a plot, and in all-sex DVDs you'll find that same variation in quality, from high-budget polish to low-budget rough edges. Many of these look like home movies, because that's what they are. The digital camera has made it possible for anyone with a little money and the right access to make and distribute a film. The medium- to low-budget DVDs will often contain extremely explicit ads for phone sex that are cheaply recycled footage from really old videos, with one come shot after another. Sometimes these ads are pretty aggressive, and contain scenes that might offend some people, such as gaping anal shots. Sometimes the immediacy of the ads' sexuality will make the films themselves seem anticlimactic; I know of several women who get so hot so fast by the shocking ads at the beginning that they claim they don't make it through the ads, masturbating to orgasm before the ads are finished!

So, with rare exceptions, the video you watch isn't going to be anything like the films you're used to viewing at the local cineplex. In terms of budget and therefore overall appearance it'll be a close, though genetically inbred, cousin of B-movies. It's also important to keep in mind that you're going to be watching a video made to feature one thing: sex. Porn makers know that the reason anyone (outside of their peers) is watching their film in the first place is to see explicit sex. So the focus in each and every film will be the sex scenes, with everything else taking a back seat.

The need to focus on sex, combined with a small budget and minimal resources, often compromises vital aspects of the video's quality. Poor sound quality and looped scenes are an unfortunate result. Sound issues can mean hearing the sounds of the production crew, muffled or inaudible dialogue, or annoying background music—sometimes, lamely enough, just music playing in the room where the actors are having sex. A huge complaint from viewers is having to sit through scenes that have been cut (often poorly) with looped film, meaning the action (such as a close-up of a blow job) is edited in repetition to make the scene seem longer. Another annoying corner-cutter found on all-sex videos is the technique of intermingling higher-quality scenes with badly filmed, lackluster scenes, for filler. As if we wouldn't notice.

NC-17 and Softcore Porn

If you're not quite ready to take the plunge, there are plenty of options that will still titillate you. You can pick a Hollywood or foreign film that has an NC-17 rating, which is essentially a soft X-rating and is either sought out by filmmakers for publicity or considered the "kiss of death" to features that hope to pull in the mainstream megabucks. Or you can choose from among European and Japanese films that enjoy fewer restrictions on sex and have a more mature, savvy viewership (not to mention legislators), so you'll find, say, French films with sex that doesn't hide—or exaggerate—real interactions between two bodies. Or you can rent a softcore feature, either a B-grade film with male and female nudity (no erections) or one with simulated sex. Or you can watch cable TV or pay-per-view porn. Cable porn is softer than "hard core"—the stuff that shows penetration—though it's very similar because these films are the edited or softened version of a fully explicit porn feature. They show no penetration or genital close-ups— but it's definitely not simulated sex!

If you want to try out some steamy Hollywood or foreign movies, try these Hollywood films:

Basic Instinct (director's cut), *Better Than Chocolate, Body of Evidence, Boogie Nights, Bound, Caligula, Crash* (director's cut), *The Fluffer, Henry and June, A History of Violence, Holy Smoke, The Hunger, Jade, Kama Sutra, Last Tango in Paris, 9 1/2 Weeks, Secretary* (highly recommended)

Foreign:
Belle du Jour, Betty Blue, Emmanuelle, Fanny Hill, Hammer horror vampire films circa 1970, *In the Realm of Passion, In the Realm of the Senses,* Lesbian vampire films by Jess Franco or Jean Rollin, *The Pillow Book, Romance, Sex and Lucia, Tokyo Decadence, The Unbearable Lightness of Being, Y tu mamá también*

why porn sucks

Porn is a fantasy world, but whose fantasy world *is* it? On the one hand, porn films appear to be made for a narrowly defined audience of single heterosexual men—all of whom like to see big-boobed blondes engaged in predictable sex acts. On the other hand, it looks like the makers of porn are trying to appeal to as many viewers as possible, with a resulting mish-mash of sexual activities.

Usually, for one reason or another, everyone has a complaint about porn. Many women (and men) feel that their sexuality isn't being truly reflected on the flickering screen. They're right—porn doesn't represent the sexual diversity we encounter in real life. Is porn sexist? Yes. Is porn racist? Yes. Porn isn't created for you, or for me—it's for that fantasy audience the producers and distributors *think* is watching porn. And most porn producers and distributors believe the audience is all white, all male, unintelligent, desperate for any kind of sexual imagery, lonely, insecure about their penis size, and possessing unrefined sexual tastes.

They're wrong. The fact is, *we're* the ones watching. And we're not just "raincoaters"—far from it, in fact. Porn is for those of us who like sex, like movies, and enjoy watching other people get off, and we're a lot more sexually sophisticated than some people think. And some of us like some of the things we see, others dislike certain things, and some of us could care less about the details. So what bothers *you*?

Porn Looks Like...Porn

When you bring home your first DVD, you may expect to see a movie just like a mega-budget Hollywood blockbuster, but one that goes "all the way" instead of fading out when the sex scene begins. I'm sorry to have to break this to you, but...porn looks like what it is. It's overlit (if lit well at all), the sets are cast-offs from *General Hospital*, the editing is sloppy, you sometimes can see boom mikes, the girls look at the camera as if they're confused (or at the director when they should be concentrating on having sex)... it's like no one checked the finished product to see if it was any good—and it's possible they didn't. In some porn films, you'll see a nearly-Hollywood standard of high production values—they even leave the lights on when the sex begins—though not all films are like this. Why not? Because outside Hollywood studios, no one has that kind of money or those resources to throw around, especially in a film genre that's controversial.

Mainstream porn is like any other film genre, with the difference that the people behind and in front of the camera usually haven't gone to school to learn and cultivate style and technique that we're used to seeing, since most folks in the industry didn't intend porn to be their first career choice. But what's truly remarkable is the large number of adult filmmakers who pull off amazing feats with virtually nothing—no budget, no time, untrained actors, and few resources. In the big business of making porn, it's the people at the top making all the distribution decisions (and all the money), while the people actually making the films—the actors, directors, and crew— are at the bottom of the money food chain. If Hollywood could do what the adult industry directors, writers, actors, and crew (and all other independent filmmakers) do out of blood, sweat, and tears, and with the same hunger to fulfill a creative drive while making a pittance, we'd have a lot more films in theaters worth watching.

Most Porn Follows a Boring Formula

This just in: everything you see on TV and in movies is based on a tried-and-true formula—porn being no exception. When a Hollywood studio makes an action film, its head honchos know that audiences expect car chases, explosions, gunfire, plenty of fighting—and the hero rescuing a pretty girl in the last shoot 'em up scene (or hopefully vice versa). Typically, though not always, genre films weave the story line around these formulaic expectations, often sacrificing character, setting, soundtrack, and filmmaking for events. You'll find the same limitations in much of mainstream porn. In a typical adult video you'll see six or seven sex scenes, including fellatio, cunnilingus, anal sex, a girl–girl scene, and lots of penis/vagina sex in doggy-style, missionary, cowgirl, and reverse cowgirl positions. The male ejaculation is almost always external, usually on the face (called a "facial"), and the sex is shown in extreme close-up. That's it. Sorry to ruin the ending for you.

Every mainstream porn video follows an unwritten rule to standardize the sex acts in a given film, and it's followed as strictly as a chemical formula to make bubble bath. This formula ensures that in each video there'll be a standard set of sex acts (blow jobs, cunnilingus, vaginal, and anal sex), positions (missionary, doggy style, reverse cowgirl) and couplings (male/female, two guys with one girl, two girls with one guy, girl–girl, and a group scene with four or more performers). Unless it's an indy, all porn follows this formula.

Apart from the standard set of positions and couplings, most porn films feature actors and actresses who are polished and coiffed to fit the ideals of Southern California–style beauty, since that's where the majority of the industry is based. An oft-voiced complaint is that the men in porn are unattractive (or look like 1980s Chippendales dancers), while the women's bodies must conform to a rigid standard of perfection: underweight, blonde hair, big lips, and big boobs (the Beverly Hills Plastic Surgery Association is always well represented).

The Indy Porn Backlash

As in Hollywood, porn has mainstream films and independent films. The term *mainstream* indicates films made by the bigger companies like Vivid, VCA, Wicked, Metro, Adam and Eve, and Evil Angel (to name a few), largely based in Southern California. Mainstream porn films are the most widely available (as they are often the darlings of the distributors), usually featuring "typical" porn actors—all stars and of little diversity in terms of skin color, ethnic background, and body size. Mainstream studios put a lot of money into their films and keep some outstanding actors and directors in their stables for years.

Independent porn, by contrast, is everyone *not* in Silicone Valley, and, as with nonadult independent movie studios, the genre has a lot of innovators and art school directors, who often are edgier and provide more realistic and thought-provoking content. Independently made porn comes from all over, though it's largely based in the United States and is made by individuals (often women) who own production companies like Burning Angel, Pink and White Productions, Maria Beatty (Bleu Productions), SIR Video and Fatale; and small companies such as Alternative Worldz, Pirate Booty Productions, Libido Films (formerly Libido Magazine), Pinkgasm, The East Van Porn Collective (Vancouver), Black Mirror Productions, and Comstock Films (New York). And there are many, many more, especially when you include the hundreds of online sex bloggers and indy paysites, phew!

With independents you'll find everything from beautiful, black-and-white, shot-on-film features to white-knuckle, gritty S/M films shot in vivid color in actual dungeons. Indy videos tend to have an overall feeling of Film School 101, but make up for any shortcomings with all the essential things that mainstream porn lacks: real couples, genuine heat and lust, sexy yet normal-looking performers, laughing, playfulness, smiles, no formula, real sex acts that regular people enjoy, full-body shots, and true enjoyment and portrayal of sex acts typically marginalized (or ridiculed) in mainstream porn.

Altporn is a genre that straddles mainstream and indy lines. This is due to the fact that websites like Suicide Girls popularized tattooed, pierced punk pinups and people wanted more (and more-explicit versions of the boys and girls they recognized from alt-subcultures). Altporn makers emerged from an online culture that fetishized the guys and gals who worked in cafés and record shops and spent their money at tattoo parlors, and started making porn—and their distaste for conventional porn made every minute of their creations worth watching. They were creative, fresh, and new, and they had a take-no-prisoners attitude about women enjoying sex and their bodies, and displayed refreshing, anti-Barbie-porn star sentiments. Mainstream porn was quick to see a cash cow on its way to the slaughterhouse and recruited a few very talented altporn directors, who make cool-looking, albeit somewhat formulaic, porn. The old

---

A Reviewer's Complaints

After years of watching porn on a daily basis for my job—as well as my personal pleasure!—I have my own list of complaints. Cookie-cutter performers and safer-sex questions aside, my axes to grind are:

- Looped and recycled footage to extend scenes
- Phone sex commercials seemingly from the 1980s
- Embarrassing grammar and spelling mistakes on DVD covers and ads
- Camera flashbulbs during sex scenes (for box cover stills)
- Hearing the director or technician when you shouldn't
- Box cover lies about content and production values
- Bad special effects
- Low DVD quality and poor DVD menus
- Assumption of a male-only audience
- Extreme, unsafe sex acts that almost exclusively exist in porn

guard of Silicone Valley has yet to treat the altporn kids (though they're mainstream funded and distributed) like equals, even though their videos outsell the "same old, same old" bimbo-driven formula porn that many studios continue to produce.

Where Are All the Hot Guys?

The short answer: in gay porn. The long answer... This is an industry that chooses women for their attractiveness, men for their "wood" (ability to get and keep an erection). Being a man in porn is not as easy as many think—it's not that you get to have sex with hot chicks all day long. You have to have an overly large penis; be able to get it up on command in front of a cast, crew, and camera; and then keep it up until someone else says you're done, which could be a very long time. At that point you have to orgasm on command, in front of everyone, probably in a difficult position—and it's best if your load is large and shoots far. And hopefully, you should be somewhat pleasant to work with. Because, after all, it's a job.

That's one reason you won't usually find hunks in porn—unless it's gay male porn. Gay men's porn is all about the hot studly men and features a more diverse selection of body types, all of whom are coincidentally hung like horses. The guys in gay male porn will range from tan, coiffed, and more muscular than your average guy—beefy but clean-looking—to sexy older men, waifish young things, and tough guys of every color. Many straight women enjoy watching gay male porn because of the way that the male body is eroticized and shown in all its sexual variety.

Straight porn lacks hunks for another reason, which may be hearsay but is widely believed: lots of folks think that the men

in straight porn are purposely selected by porn makers to be
less attractive than your average guy. The belief is that hot hunks
will intimidate the male viewer, and that watching a good-look-
ing star with the fantasy woman onscreen would bruise his ego.
This way, the male viewer's ego stays intact. To me this is illog-
ical; would action films be easier for men to watch if the heroes
were purposely ugly? I doubt it.

Besides the unusual physical qualifications of the male porn
star, the other fact remains that many of the men in porn have
gotten onscreen by being in the right place at the right time—
with an easily controlled erection. There are lots of attractive
men coming into the business these days. If you don't find a male
star who appeals to you, keep looking, and check out different
genres and eras. Some porn has no men at all, and some features
men only as props. For instance, in many Andrew Blake films
you often won't even see the male actors' heads or faces, just
their lower bodies!

The Performers Look Like They're Going Through the Motions

They probably are. Porn is a job like any other, and it often shows
in lame, boring sex scenes where the performers don't even make
eye contact. If this happens to you, turn off the video and get
another one. Write an irritated review on a site like Adult DVD
Talk, where many porn directors, actors, and even producers
are members, and will likely read every post that contains their
names. You don't have to settle for mediocre porn with uninter-
ested actors. Unfortunately, because porn is made on limited
budgets and porn performers need to make lots of movies to

earn a living, many bored-looking people end up in videos around the world. Not all videos are like that, however, and oodles of movies show people who really can't keep their hands off each other. Porn with chemistry that sizzles sells well, and pornographers are waking up to this fact, being motivated to feature more, and more honestly hot, scenes in their films.

The work of indy directors is a great place to find lots of heat, and amateur porn with its unscripted nature, as well as European films, all typically pack genuine lust and unrushed eroticism. While many mainstream porn directors have great films but cold sex scenes, a few directors (John Leslie being one) shoot scenes that could burn a hole through your screen. Some mainstream porn films even have real-life couples. The *Deep Inside* series focuses on an actress's favorite scenes—and you can see why these are her favorites, some even showcasing a scene where the actress has sex with someone she loves.

Porn Music Sucks, Too

Yes, it does. Bad music ruins a good sex scene, and in fact music in general, if it's not to your taste, can be too distracting. Many of the all-sex, no-plot directors don't use music of any kind, featuring the natural sounds of the actors having sex (Christoph Clark is a great example). Unfortunately, some will try to dress up a video or correct spoiled sound with music that is *their* idea of sexy—usually not yours. If you get a video with irritating music but great visuals, turn the sound down, or off. Play your own music if you want.

In porn, when the action begins, they usually cue a wholly different type of music, music sure to dampen any prior arousal the viewer has cultivated, a sort of audio anaphrodisiac. Bad porn music is like an embarrassing side effect of a promising arousal pill, and is part and parcel of our porn-viewing experience. Most porn consumers hate it (and most porn reviewers loathe it), yet we're stuck with it during some pretty crucial masturbatory moments, and we either put up with it or consign ourselves to the "mute" button.

Movie music is an art. Porn is seldom art, so it's no surprise that most porn music is awful. Movie music is seldom done well either, but in regular nonerotic films, the person (or team) doing the scoring takes into account a variety of factors with the goal of enhancing the feeling, mood, or action onscreen. Perhaps porn scorers believe they're doing the same when they slap that wa-wa, wokka-wokka, or wailing rock guitar track over the same old sex scenes. Porn films are by no means the same as Hollywood films, and perhaps shouldn't be put to the same types of music, but many of us who dread music that often ruins our horniness think that more effort should be put into the aural atmosphere elicited by porn's auteurs.

Movie music that works well goes largely unnoticed by the rapt viewer, but still subtly manipulates the feelings inspired by the filmmaker's images and narrative. It adds to the creepiness of a David Lynch film or takes you into dreamy worlds crafted by Danny Elfman. Bad music interrupts the scene, distracts from the story (usually by trying to be showy or too hip), or gives away the impending danger (Freddy, Jason, et al.).

In porn we have a whole different ball of wax—porn music by nature must be different than the type of movie music we're used to, because generally we watch porn for an entirely different reason: to get off. Porn seldom has a watchable plot, and

because decent plot in porn seems so fragile, elusive, and shak-
ily held together when you do find it, the music seems as if it
would be just another thing that can go wrong. So unless the
porn video is going to have a professional treatment on all levels,
we can only assume that a good score is going to be hard to
find, because you have to score not only an actual film but also
one with the unusual element of extended scenes of explicit
sex, intended for masturbatory gratification. This is something
that Hollywood pros have no experience with, either, though
it would be interesting to see what concept Angelo Badalamenti
would come up with.

Porn without plot is sometimes put to music. Such wall-to-
wall films, where the sex scenes take place in their own world
and the scenes are loosely strung together by a theme, are typically the most egregious offenders of bad music put to sex.
Gonzo films, where the cameraman directs and participates in
the scene, resulting in a first-person experience, rarely ever have
music in them—thus lending the reality porn feel. Maybe this
is why I've become such a fan of gonzo porn lately, because nothing is worse than awful music when I want to lose myself in
fantasy onscreen sex, and when porn is shot sans music, I get
to hear the real, natural sounds of sex (an incredible turn-on).

They Never Show S/M with Sex

But wait a minute—BDSM is a sexual practice, and porn is about
sex, so why don't they show the two together? Those who practice and play with S/M know how hot and sexy these two great
tastes are together, and renting an S/M video with sexy players who do nothing more than lamely spank each other in

faux-S/M outfits can be pretty disappointing. Unfortunately, in the eyes of the law, anything outside of vanilla sex is considered edgy content—even though many regular people engage in nonvanilla sex every day. The problem is, many lawmakers believe that S/M and sexual practices such as fisting are harmful—they simply don't understand what these practices really are. And, contrary to what the lawmakers think, S/M *isn't* about abuse, degradation, or nonconsensual violation, such as rape.

In reality, the sensual rituals and games that fall under "S/M" are for people who love, respect, and trust one another. When a couple engages in S/M, they experience the thrill, rush, and arousal that come from an agreed-upon exchange of power. One lover holds down her sweetheart's hands while she administers loving spanks to his naughty, gleefully wriggling behind; two lovers dress in leather, lingerie, or uniforms and play erotic games of dominance and submission with sexual rewards; one partner enjoys surrendering to the feeling of restraint and allows herself to be sensually whipped into erotic bliss that can only come from surrender, fantasy fulfillment, and intense physical stimulation. Sex and S/M in combination can make for the most unforgettable, mind-blowing, pivotal, emotional, and even spiritual sexual experiences imaginable.

The state of the law in the United States about sexually explicit material revolves around keeping pornographers and adult retailers on their toes, never knowing for what, or when, they might be prosecuted for offending community standards. You see, the law in this country states that something is considered obscene, and therefore illegal to create or distribute, if a court somewhere says it is. You might hear people in and out of the adult industry say things like "Showing urination is illegal," or "Showing S/M with sex is illegal," or "Portraying Bill O'Reilly as a journalist is illegal" (and if isn't, it should be)—and all these cautious statements are incorrect. In fact, there's only a single test, which is when a court in any of the fifty states decides that a particular thing (DVD, book, picture, fake journalist, whatever) is, by the "standards of the community," obscene.

No one making S/M porn knows whether what they're doing is illegal or not. That is, until they receive a sweet invitation called an "indictment" and attend a party just for them called a "trial," followed by a big hangover called a "conviction." Then they've been (albeit arbitrarily) bad. This situation, reminiscent of organized crime tactics, is not an oversight; the U.S. Supreme Court is well aware that the only way that retailers and pornographers can really be sure they won't be prosecuted for selling obscene material is for them to avoid portraying activities that might possibly be interpreted as obscene—*anywhere*. So meanwhile, the courts seem smug and pleased with themselves, conservative politicians can trot out a pet cause when the polls are flagging, and the retailers and creators of the most widely recognized product (outside the 99-cent hamburger) in America sweat through every single business day—while the government never actually makes smut categorically illegal.

In a court case for obscenity, the accused is held to whatever the local community's standards are for obscenity, as determined by a jury. The real question is, whose morality or virtue is being offended here? That of a jury sitting there worrying about how much work they're missing while stuck in court? That of the many people who bought or rented the DVD? And whose community standards come into question when you're talking about a consumer product? Former Attorney General John Ashcroft found the exposed breast of a statue (lady justice herself) in the halls of our own Justice Department to be obscene, and ordered it covered up at the cost of $8,000 in our tax dollars. *I* found the one-million-dollar per episode salary for each cast member of *Friends* to be obscene (that was twenty-two episodes per season, folks). But an act of mutual sexual pleasure between adults? Please—spare me, *and* my tax dollars.

Bottom line: legality and porn are a big crapshoot for retailers and pornographers. In many cases, producers have decided to avoid material that could cause problems, though some are willing to take a chance and portray sexuality in a more diverse and realistic light, and are ready to face the consequences. In my opinion, I say let the consumers decide—keep the courts out of it.

chapter 5

find the right porn for you

Finding the DVD, streaming video, or porn site that turns you on and gets you off is no easy proposition, even if you already know what you want to see. Porn is a vast genre with many subgenres, full of its own language and customs, confusing labels, and misleading titles—plus a whole lot of bad grammar. What's worse, many retailers (online and off) treat their stock with carelessness or even distaste, cramming porn together with no discernable sense of order. Alphabetical order is not invited to the party, Dewy decimal has left the building. And each website seems to have its own organizational logic. It would make a librarian homicidal. Even a naughty one.

In a lot of ways, finding the right porn is much like seeking out a Hollywood movie—you're really on your own to find it. But in a genre of film that has no road map, you'll need to know not only what you want and where to find it, but also the different types of porn available.

Start by creating a picture of what you hope to find in your porn, just as you'd order a meal in a restaurant. What are you hungry for? Small breasts, big butts, women in charge, realistic plots, blow jobs, two gals and a guy, male anal penetration, rough sex? This may not be *your* menu, but you get the idea. The important thing is that you make a list of all the qualities you hope to find in an adult video. Then make a second list of things you *don't* want to see. Do you get turned off by fake breasts, hairy men, rimming, toe-sucking, facial ejaculation, two women together, or watching group sex? These are just examples to get you brainstorming about what you think will send you over the edge—and what you think you'll want to skip through. As you watch porn, you'll probably find more to add to (or subtract from) either list, because sometimes we find things that turn us on or off that we didn't even know about.

For instance, you might want a DVD with no plot, all-natural women, authentic female orgasms, and no men. Or maybe you want a great story line and believable acting, and you don't care what anyone looks like as long as the sex is hot. Perhaps you want an S/M film that looks beautiful, with no plot and with real couples. Maybe you want a lesbian love story but no genital close-ups. You might be fantasizing about a specific type of story, where the women are the main focus, but you don't want anal penetration. Or you want all-anal, as rough as it gets.

Avoiding What You Don't Like

You can avoid seeing sexual images or activities that you don't want to see, though some things, like facial ejaculation and anal sex, are practically in every video. It will help to be aware of your own expectations. Be prepared for the inevitable: no matter how open-minded you are, you will at some point come across a DVD cover, promo photo, turn of phrase, or scene in porn that will offend you. Just because it's out there doesn't mean you ever have to have it in your life for more than that fleeting instant. Know what you *don't* like—this will help you make a selection that won't leave you high and dry or, in the worst-case scenario, angry or disgusted.

Knowing what you like and dislike before you even begin your search can help enormously. You can single out many of your preferences before you rent or buy, and then skip the parts you don't care for. Consumer reviews on online porn websites (explained at the end of this chapter) are very helpful in these matters. The reviews and ratings can also help you select videos where you can see things you don't usually witness on the blue screen, such as an all-natural cast (that is, actresses without breast implants), internal ejaculation, attention to cinematography and lighting, great acting, and excellent plot.

As a general rule, most women-owned sex toy stores never carry films that are demeaning or abusive toward women or that contain racist or discriminatory content—of any kind. They often have complicated screening procedures that make sure their porn portrays healthy sexuality, meaning that the videos depict positive attitudes about sex (no sexual shame allowed!), and show women getting off as much as the men. Such videos always pay attention to female pleasure. The porn these shops carry won't model unsafe sex practices, such as inserting anything anally that can get "lost" in the rectum. Whenever something borderline or potentially button-pressing comes up in a video with an overwhelming redeeming quality, such as a standout sex scene or underrepresented content, the store owners often make sure that their product descriptions warn customers about it.

What's on the Box

When you're considering a DVD, look closely at the back and front covers, or any promo photos. Check for the names you want to see, or for ones you want to avoid. Look at the teeny-tiny pictures—these will be stills taken during filming. You can see right off the bat if there's anything you don't like. Sometimes you'll see pictures of scenes or actresses that aren't in the video, though this is happening less frequently as consumer outcry makes pornographers begin to guarantee that images on the covers actually come from the video itself. By all means, don't get a video with an offensive title, subtitle, or image. Get a DVD you'll feel okay about watching, whether or not you get off.

Box covers in porn are glossy, colorful, and very eye-catching—and usually sexually explicit. Higher-budget films will have a big, fancy, professionally retouched photo on the front cover, with the star or stars looking *way* better than they will in the

What the Hell Is a "Reverse Cowgirl"?

The adult industry might as well be its own country. It has its own strange customs—and its own language. Over the years, a lexicon has evolved out of slang, nicknames, and verbal shortcuts to comprise a whole world of terminology. Terms such as *wood, reverse cowgirl, DP, pro-am,* and *suitcase pimp* all describe specific body parts, positions, sex acts, film subgenres, and the types of characters you'd find on or around a porn set. Just as the locals in a surf town (or skate culture, or BMX culture) have their own lingo, the porn industry takes the terms for granted and uses them as if everyone knew what they meant. You'll find them on box covers, in industry magazines, and in interviews with performers.

actual film. All-sex features have a couple of collaged images on the cover, as a sample of the performers inside (usually the more conventionally beautiful ones), with small images of the explicit action around them as window dressing. These small images might be slightly censored or nonexplicit. Other genres will have a range of covers, from the high-budget style (looks like an ordinary movie) to the low budget (cramming in as many pics as possible). The back covers will have many more tiny explicit photos—look at these eye-straining photos closely, and you'll have a pretty good idea of what's in the video. In the high-budget features, the layout might be more like a regular movie box, with a small descriptive blurb about the feature and the sex acts and perhaps a short review or endorsement from an adult video magazine or website.

The text on the box covers will range from hilarious to offensive, from artsy to unintelligible and error-ridden. The words can be so misspelled and ungrammatical that you won't know whether you want to laugh or weep openly for the public school system. Still, the description, however haphazard, will give you an idea about what you'll find inside. In all-sex films, it's a good idea either to look for porn that states that all its box cover images depict scenes on the video (your seal of approval), or to stick with reputable companies or directors. For quality in features, look for well-known production houses, directors, and stars.

Accolades for Porn Films?

A video is more likely to have something in it worth watching if it has won any awards or honors such as high reviews from sites like Adult DVD Talk, or awards from *AVN (Adult Video News)*,

Smart Girl's Porn Vocabulary

Bukkake: A group of men gather around and ejaculate onto a woman. Where the ejaculations end up depends on the filmmaker: face, whole body, mouth—in one film, the actress wears a dog cone.

Cream Pie: An actress with come visibly dripping from her vagina or anus.

DP (Double Penetration): Two men penetrating one woman in the ass and the vagina at the same time. (In gay porn, two men penetrating one man in the ass simultaneously.)

FIP (Fake Internal Pop Shot): The cable version of an orgasmic climax in which both partners simply shudder violently, faking orgasm.

Fluffer: A woman or man used to stimulate male talent through oral sex before they go on camera.

Gape, Gapes, Gaping: Term for when the pussy or ass is stretched or held open to create a hole you can see into. Currently a trendy fetish in the all-sex genre.

Money Shot: Male ejaculation captured on film; volume and distance are highly prized.

Pearl Necklace: Term referring to ejaculation onto a woman's neckline and breasts, thereby simulating a string of pearls.

Pop Shot: When a man ejaculates, and it's caught on film.

Reverse Cowgirl: Woman on top, facing away from man while having sex, ideal for spread-wide angles because it provides the maximum view of penetration.

Snowballing: The term for swapping ejaculate from one mouth to anther, or kissing someone after they've received a mouthful of come. Also called *come swapping.*

Hot d'Or, *Adam Film World*, or XRCO Choice (X-Rated Critics Organization). *AVN* magazine and *Hot Video* magazine both produce yearly awards events that bestow honors on worthy videos, crew, directors, and actors. Each of the events is a lavish production—big money, black-tie, haute couture, limo-packed. At these well-attended spectacles big stars show lots of the skin you've grown to know and love in their videos, and plenty of lone guys flock to ogle and have their pictures taken with the stars in the event's off-hours. The awards ceremonies themselves are steeped in tradition, last for ages, and serve dinner to the esteemed guests who paid hundreds of dollars a seat.

AVN is a magazine by and for the porn industry (*not* for the consumer, as you'll glean by the highly industry-specific porn tastes revealed in its reviews). The scope of *AVN* is fairly wide-ranging, including everything from movie reviews by genre to free speech news and legal updates on American porn censorship. It's a slick, glossy magazine full of ads for the latest releases; industry gossip; news about stars, directors, and production houses; and selected (though pro-porn industry, anti-everyone else) reviews of porn, adult books, comics, magazines, sex toys, S/M gear, and adult websites. *AVN* has a sprawling site, avn.com (beware of a pop-up), and spin-off magazines such as *AVN Online*. Every year in Las Vegas it holds an awards event and convention for the porn industry; indy porn filmmakers are seldom, if ever, included in the awards.

There, their juries select from industry-nominated films a whole roster of nepotistic winners for a variety of categories, ranging from Best New Starlet and Best Director to Best Fellatio Scene. Winning an award is a coveted prize, and can launch careers, boost sales, and make a film noticed by everyone. When you see an *AVN* award or nomination, at least you know the film is worth watching. *AVN* also has an all-gay-male version, the GayVN's. *AVN* also awards a Best European Film honor called the AVN d'Or.

The Palme d'Or is the highest award possible for a director to receive at Cannes, the celebrated international film festival conducted yearly in France. Held at the same time as Cannes, the Hot d'Or Awards celebrate European adult films, much like the *AVNs*. Produced by French magazine *Hot Video*, often called the French version of *AVN*, the event packs more than 500 people into a ballroom every year. They give a nod to America's mainstream porn industry with selective awards—though usually the general contenders for awards are half American, half European. In the jury process, few awards are actually selected by industry professionals—called the Professional Vote—and most are selected by *Hot Video*'s readers.

The XRCO (X-Rated Critics Association) Awards are held every year in Century City, California. These awards are voted on by members of the mainstream adult media, and though the ceremonies are much smaller and intimate, with little of the nonindustry throngs that clog up events like *AVN*'s, the event is still piled high with porneratti glitz and glam. The XRCO is composed of mainstream porn critics and reviewers from adult publications that include *Adam Film World*, *AVN*, and *Hustler*, as well as related Internet retail sites. *Adam Film World Guide* is an industry magazine that serves as a guide and hosts a readers' poll to select the award winners.

Many other erotic film festivals flourish around the world, such as the Barcelona Erotic Film Festival, the 18 Awards (in the U.K.), the New York City Erotic Film Fest, Hump! in Seattle (exclusively for indies), and more. Some independent adult films occasionally cause a stir at nonerotic independent film festivals, as did Maria Beatty's *The Black Glove.*

The Name Says It All

Porn titles will make you laugh or cry, arouse you or make you want to run away screaming—sometimes all at once. The desperate namers try every possible crass (and clever) deviation on any remotely sexual saying, phrase, or nonerotic movie title. Although the titles can seem simultaneously idiotic, amusing, salacious, lowbrow, and lame, what the porn is called can actually tell you quite a lot about what you're about to watch.

Many serial videos have no plot, and the title will tell you the main theme of the series. The obvious ones focus on a particular sex act, such as *Real Female Masturbation, Gush, Buttman's Big Tit Adventure, Blowjob Fantasies, Bend Over Boyfriend*—the list runs to infinity. Some series titles include a name that denotes a particular director's style, like Shane, Seymore Butts, Ben Dover, Ed Powers, and others. Many offer a stylistic theme, such as a film style, concept, or gimmick. The *Voyeur* series, for example, is seen through the eyes of a mysterious peeping tom and is the product of a single director, John Leslie.

Feature porn, or porn with a plot (often a *very* loose term), will have names that are all over the map. The name depends on what the filmmaker wants to convey, and how much he cares—or doesn't care—about the product and the viewer. It should be noted, however, that the majority of pornographers don't seem to consider their audience to be very smart and think they're catering to—or making fun of—an uneducated, unsophisticated viewer who provides their bread and butter. On the flipside, many directors and producers do care about the end product as a living legacy, a video that will be seen by all types of people, and will therefore strive to make complete, even artistic films. One obstacle in porn is that it's tough to make a fully realized film when you have to include the same specific scenes in each video. Nonetheless, like the classics, features will have a variety of names: movie-like, smart, evocative, romantic, dumb, or hilarious.

Buffy the Vampire Layer

While I can't vouch for the film quality of these titles, here's a sampling of some great adult spoof titles:

Ally McFeal	*Juranal Park*
American Booty	*Moulin Splooge*
The Bare Dick Project	*The Ozporns*
Blowjob Impossible	*Pimped by an Angel*
Buffy the Vampire Layer	*Poltergash*
Cliffbanger	*Saturday Night Beaver*
A Clockwork Orgy	*Shaving Ryan's Privates*
Das Boob	*Snatch Adams*
Dude, Where's My Dildo?	*The Sopornos*
Edward Penishands	*A Tale of Two Titties*
Ejacula	*Thighs Wide Open*
Fast Times at Deep Crack High	*Thunderboobs*
Free Will Humping	*Twin Cheeks*
Honey, I Blew Everybody	*White Men Can't Hump*
Howard Sperm's Private Parties	

Spoofs of mainstream movies or cult classics are the best-known titles in porn culture, and sometimes they're really good spoofs. Usually, though, they're just a long running joke that never gets off the ground, and all you have is a porn film with actors trying to say lines with bad accents in costumes that would make a drag queen want to claw her own eyes out.

Finding what you want to see is still going to be something of a trial-and-error process, and you'll need to be open to the fact that you're on an ongoing, exciting search for hot porn. Your ideas and fantasies will become refined and shaped as you discover what sex acts you like, what type of performers you enjoy, and how you prefer to see them presented. Because our desires and fantasies are constantly changing, no one model of porn—such as all-sex or plot-only—is going to fulfill every visual fantasy you have at every period of your life. And because finding specific titles, directors, and actors is a constant challenge in a genre that's haphazardly maintained by retailers, you'll need to have a number of alternate choices ready when you get your wallet out.

Online Reviews and Porn Communities

Besides getting recommendations from friends and suggestions from women-friendly porn retailers, your best bet for finding good porn, or at least porn with a few wank-worthy scenes, is through online review and porn community resources. Sites like Free-association.net, Friendster.com, and Orkut.com are called "social networking" sites: members-only sites where people join groups and learn more about their interests, from travel to sex and beyond—making the porn groups a great resource for honest

consumer opinion and discussion. Plus, you can join them relatively anonymously (age restrictions always apply for adult
groups) and feel confident about asking questions and partic-
ipating in discussions without anyone knowing more about
you than you'd like.

There are a significant number of message board and discussion sites that pertain exclusively to porn, outside the social
networking strata. Sites like AdultDVDTalk.com feature thousands of consumer reviews and a vibrant, alive online community
that keeps up with new releases, porn gossip, and more. This
sounds like an ad, which it's not, but I heartily endorse Adult
DVD Talk because the forums are mostly moderated by women;
they feature reviews by, for, and geared toward women; and,
unlike the point of view held by some in the porn industry, they
know that women don't want anything dumbed down or softened for their gender. This site also has a lot of members who
are porn performers (some big-name stars regularly jump into
forum discussions), and a healthy handful of porn directors
and filmmakers participate as well, so it's a great place to voice
opinions and have them heard.

But it's really ADVDT's rabid review system that's the most
useful tool for our purposes; you can count on several different
reviews from very different perspectives on a single DVD—
immensely helpful for shopping. Do keep in mind that, as with
any other discussion forum about porn, you'll occasionally
encounter things (opinions, terminology, points of view) that
you might find offensive, though the proactive moderators are
excellent about policing abusive members. But if there's something in porn you'd rather not see or find distasteful I promise
you'll find at least a few fans of it in the forums, so forewarned

is forearmed. There are a number of other porn forums and personal review sites (like RogReviews.com), and this one may lead to others you like better; Adult DVD Talk just happens to be my favorite.

Another route for consumer reviews is to visit porn rental and retail sites that post customer reviews, though of course they always reflect the taste (or lack thereof) of the individual reviewer. And not all sites will have honest reviews; some are staff-written to sell product, so turn on your bullshit detector and read through several reviews on different DVDs before you believe what you read. If it seems like they're all written by the same person, if the reviews don't really explain what's in the DVD (can you tell if they *really* watched it?), or if there are no negative reviews, be very cautious about believing the write-ups. Also, try to stick with reputable retailers that present consumer reviews, sites like AdamEve.com, AdultDVDEmpire.com, Amazon.com (yes, they sell some porn), SugarDVD.com, BlueDoor.com, XRentDVD.com, FlickSmart.com, WantedList.com, and the terrific women-centric combo site ForTheGirls.com. You can also find out a great deal about titles not by browsing consumer reviews, but by visiting retail sites that individually review their DVDs, rather than just regurgitating box cover copy or promo text. Some sites that sell porn and write about it themselves are Babeland.com, Blowfish.com, ComeAsYouAre.com, GoodVibes.com, and Libida.com.

porn's anatomy

In general, you'll find that all porn can be grouped into general categories that are widely used by trade magazines, video retailers, and others in the industry. By and large, these groupings are fairly contrived, based on antiquated notions of what distributors (the old boys' network) think male viewers want to see. You might not find all these categories in your search, or you might find even more than what's listed here—though there's no uniform method for describing porn, and your searching might take you through some haphazard methods of categorization.

Bisexual

Bi porn is always in demand, and when it's hot, it sizzles. However, generally budgets on bi videos are low, and the sex is often lackluster. It could be that the gay male actors are playing "bi for pay," that directors are being homophobic about the material, or simply that the low budgets aren't making anyone smile. In fact, the mainstream porn industry is so rife with homophobia (and perceptions of viewers' homophobia) that bi porn is often relegated to freak, or fetish, categories despite the genre's pop-ularity. Still, you can find a few gems here and there, especially from independents cashing in on the high bi demand.

Bisexuality, by definition, is sexual attraction to both men and women. So you'd think that bisexual films would show women with women, then men with men, and at some point everybody all together, like a sexually explicit version of *Bob and Carol and Ted and Alice*. But in porn, it's taken for granted that all the women have sex with each other for work, and they're not lesbians, so no one considers them bisexual. Hmmm. So it seems that bisexual films must mean those that show two men having sex together but now and then going for a woman, or women. But the funny thing is, all bi films, with few exceptions, are made with gay male performers...so I guess the gay men are the bisexual ones, swingin' with women for pay. Confused yet?

Well, I promise that you won't get too hung up on definitions when you see the unhinged lust that occurs in the boy–boy–girl three-way scenes—which are the *raison d'être* of the bisexual genre. There's a reason that this type of porn is so in demand, and it's that when it's done right, it's red-hot. This is what the Roman orgies, and the ecstatic sexuality of truly decadent debauchery through history, were really about—men and women crawling all over each other, not caring about who or what, with no hang-ups, just wanting to give and get as much pleasure as possible. Many people fantasize about two men screwing one woman (or more), and yet find it difficult to locate porn that's honest about the fact that *all these people are willingly having sex with each other*—and in the process deliciously, deliberately breaking all taboos. Yet it's entirely possible in the realm of bisexual porn.

Not all bisexual porn is created equal, of course, not by a long shot. Straight porn is extremely homophobic: its hallmark features two men (or more) having sex with one woman, while desperately trying not to touch, or look at, or be aroused by each other (often painfully obvious and distracting, I might add). Conversely, bisexual films tend to be created with a certain distaste for the material and as a result suffer in many ways. The filmmakers of bisexual material seem confused about who the audience is, and performances are generally robotic and lack-luster owing to poor casting and lack of directorial enthusiasm. And all too many bisexual videos feature two gay performers having sex with each other while desperately trying not to enjoy the female participants.

However, some performers and directors do see the erotic potential in bisexual porn and make incredible videos. They're out there, I promise. Finding them isn't easy, and you'll need to do a bit of hit-and-miss exploration until you find performers and directors you like. Look for European productions (many will come from the Czech Republic) that feature amateur performers who tend to approach bisexuality without the sexual hang-ups of their American counterparts and deliver energetic, authentic scenes. Domestic directors vary greatly, and if you like the polished look of gay performers and female porn stars and want a professional finish on your bi films, look for videos directed by ChiChi LaRue. Female performer Tina Tyler has been a bisexual activist within the porn industry for many years, and her bi films always have several sizzling, truly enthusiastic scenes in them—where even though it's obvious she's having sex with gay men, they really, truly look like they're having a lot of fun with Tina.

Classics

"Classic" or "Golden Age" porn embraces adult videos made in the 1970s and '80s. This term is also used when a particular film or video has a cultural or social significance, is notorious for one or more reasons, or has become a cult or underground favorite, such as *Deep Throat, Debbie Does Dallas,* or *The Devil in Miss Jones.* Almost every film in this category was shot using film stock, for the traditional camera technology, of course, predates the now-widespread use of digital cameras, DVDs, and even VCRs and computers. The real film stock gives these films a more movie-like feel and quality and, except for the nudity and explicit sex, makes them often indistinguishable from Hollywood films released at the same time.

It's not just the film stock that makes these films different and a cut above the rest in movie-making terms, for porn made twenty-plus years ago was a whole different animal. Each feature was created to be projected onto a big screen in a movie theater, and more care was given to make a complete film. Plots were complex, actors were skilled and remarkable, and showing explicit sex was dealt with as an exciting taboo—one that performers were delighted to explore and enthusiastic to break.

By the late 1960s, however, adult movies had settled comfortably into adult movie houses. These were old theaters that exclusively showed pornographic films, usually all day and evening long. The audience was primarily thought to be "raincoaters": men who slinked into the theaters to masturbate, though occasionally women and couples ventured in to do pretty much the same thing as the single guys. Hilariously (or sadly), modern pornographers still think their viewership is composed of these raincoaters—a very telling sign of the age of the people still making the decisions in mainstream porn. Porn was also watched at home on movie projectors or at smokers or stag parties— gatherings attended by single or married men, with no women. When *Deep Throat* was released, the attention it received sent regular Americans into the adult theaters in droves. Much of the attention came when bad-boy heartthrob Frank Sinatra used his own in-home movie projector in a private screening for Vice President Spiro Agnew.

An understanding of the culture at the time these films were made is crucial to appreciating the milieu of classic porn and its modern counterparts. In the early 1970s the industry was on the cusp of an explosion, reveling in the fact that adult films were being made by people who thought their work championed the free-speech provisions of the First Amendment to the Constitution. This attitude was likely being fueled by the lifting of the archaic Motion Picture Production Code in 1968, and the subsequent release of Hollywood films containing previously taboo themes (like *Rosemary's Baby*, 1968) and sometimes a lot less clothing (such as *Barbarella*, also 1968). Porn actor Richard Pacheco soberingly adds that his generation at this time had a "take a pill mentality" about everything from syphilis to unwanted pregnancy. This was the beginning of the 1970s, and while Barbarella could bare her boobs and have orgasms in outer space, being involved in a porn film could get you convicted for pimping and pandering, a three-year-imprisonment felony offense. Everyone who participated in adult films at this time stuck together. They'd meet at restaurants and move to undisclosed locations for shooting.

Beauty standards as seen in popular culture were different then: Makeup, hair, and clothes were worn differently; shaving and waxing body hair weren't yet trends; and surgical augmentation was rare. The subject matter sometimes followed along taboo lines that today's filmmakers—both adult and nonerotic—wouldn't dare explore. Staying true to plot and character, directors depicted explicit violence right alongside the sex, something you'd never see in today's cautious adult features. Incest, rape, and loss of virginity were not-uncommon themes, and entire features such as the famous *Behind the Green Door* were about women who were kidnapped and forced into sexual servitude. These films were far from politically correct—racial stereotypes were prevalent and female characters were often coerced into nonconsensual sexual situations.

All the same, you can find classic porn with no taboo themes whatsoever, such as elaborate musicals, with song, dance, great costumes—*and* hot sex. Or thoughtful, intense explorations of relationships, with emotions running the gamut of human expression. Films could be goofy, fun, and light, but could turn dirty and explicit as viewers followed the exploits of giggling cheerleaders (*Debbie Does Dallas*), desperately horny hospital workers (*Candy Stripers*), or sexually demanding housewives (*Outlaw Ladies*). Also, the line between porn and Hollywood cinema became blurred for a short period, producing films such as *Caligula*, as well as cult crossover hits like *Café Flesh*.

Just as with any film, each classic bears the individual stamp of the director. Direction style, cinematography, editing, the way script and plot were communicated to the viewer, and the performance of the actors all depended on the vision and synthesis of the director's overall concept for the film. This was especially true in classic porn, where these things were prized highly. Also, because feature-length porn was in its fledgling stage, directors from porn's Golden Age often came from film backgrounds or worked in the film industry, whereas now porn directors often learn film from within porn but have little outside film experience. Classic porn directors not only possessed well-rounded film experience, such as Robert McCallum (who worked as Orson Welles's cameraman for fifteen years), but also cited a variety of artistic influences on their work, such as Radley Metzger (aka Henry Paris), who was heavily influenced by French art-house directors like Buñuel and Bergman.

Educational

Videos in the educational category typically have some instructional or informative content but also feature explicit demonstrations of sex. They can cover topics such as female ejaculation, male masturbation, learning S/M negotiation and techniques, or having sex with someone with spinal-cord injury—to name just a few. Some companies have large catalogs and lengthy title lists, with several series tapes on particular subjects, such as sex and aging, or positions. A number of porn stars have decided to show the world exactly how the pros do it, and their videos feature lessons on techniques, followed by demonstrations. Nina Hartley's many educational tapes showcase her training as a nurse as well as a porn actress and are excellent at delivering information. Many people like educational tapes because some show real couples having sex, often for the first time in front of a camera.

Videos that educate sexually offer a wealth of information on sexual health and pleasure, in a variety of contexts, on a wide range of topics, and focus on individual sexual preferences and orientations. You can learn female anatomy for pleasure—not reproduction—or how to give a man an erotic massage that will blow his mind. You can watch real-life couples demonstrate sexual positions that offer a variety of sexual benefits, while you're learning and being titillated at the same time. Or you can get a hands-on tour of sex toys, or a lesson on making love to women given by porn stars. There are how-to tapes on oral sex, anal sex, erotic massage, swinging, bondage, and discipline—you name it, and it's out there on tape. And if you haven't thought of it, some erstwhile sex educator is probably working on it right now.

You can use sexual how-to videos in a variety of ways to enhance your sex life. Simply watching an erotic video can give you new ideas, strategies, or knowledge that you can put into practice to improve sex whether solo or partnered. Most of these videos contain explicit sex and follow a formula of part education, part arousal, with demonstrations intended to turn on viewers so they'll want to try the techniques right away. Watching a sex ed DVD with your lover—as a lark, as a serious learning experience, or just for fun—can get you both turned on, give you fuel for new adventures, or introduce a new idea, such as trying oral or anal sex or a new position. Plus, watching a new technique and seeing how it's done is often easier and less anxiety provoking than reading about it in a book or having someone describe it to you.

Not all sex ed DVDs are created equal. Many contain bits of inaccurate information or make unfair judgments about other people's sexual practices. Because some education tapes are made by entrepreneurs, rather than trained sex educators, they can contain unsafe information as well. *Viewer beware.*

Sometimes the quality of the information is high, yet typically little money is put into sex ed tapes, so production values and budgets are usually (though not always) low. The result is that many homemade-feeling videos are usually taped in one setting, though some with higher budgets will be shot in various locations. Many from the bigger production houses will have a talking head—a sex educator/narrator who introduces the material and guides viewers through the scenes. The strange thing about sex ed videos is that they all feel really dated—even many made just a few years ago seem to have a 1980s feel. Consider yourself warned about big hair.

European

Porn from Europe is a much-loved thing, filmed in beautiful locations, with great visual film techniques, high budgets, and plenty of gorgeous European actors. Most European adult performers are very different in appearance from their Silicone Valley (read: surgically enhanced) counterparts, and their approach to sex is refreshingly open, playful, and unrushed. Often, the women exhibit their lusty sexuality in a way that comes across as more earthy and genuine than that of many American performers, while the men actually take the time to enjoy the women they're with. Unfortunately, sound quality is often poor or the dialogue is badly dubbed (if at all). Many American directors travel to Eastern Europe to take advantage of the lovely locations, low costs, and enthusiastic talent, and we all benefit when they do. While some European films are made in England, France, Italy, Czech Republic (principally in Prague), and Spain, most of them are filmed in and around Budapest, Hungary, the European equivalent of Southern California's porn epicenter

Features

This large and unwieldy category includes all porn containing a plot, whether shot on film stock or on digital video (DV). You'll find incredible, full-length movies in this category, made by a whole roster of talented directors who are interesting and eccentric in the way they create movies. Each director has his or her own style. This is where you'll find erotic comedies, drama, crime films, love stories, and film noir. Quite a few of these films are groomed for what the industry calls the couples market—pairs of men and women watching together.

Features are released both by big studios and by independent artists. Big studios, such as Evil Angel, VCA, Vivid, Wicked, and Metro, will have high-budget, polished feature films that use porn stars and employ the standard formula for sex scenes. They contract with in-house directors, who each have their own style. In choosing a good feature, what matters isn't the name of the studio, but rather the name of the director who makes the kinds of films *you* like. Certain feature-directors take themselves seriously as filmmakers and create films for an audience they believe to be connoisseurs of both porn and film. Some directors make great films that parody adult filmmaking or the adult industry experience—intended for an industry-savvy audience. A few feature-directors are simply trying to make a buck, creating porn with a plot for a variety of reasons, usually because their producer wants porn for the couples market—soft-focus, romantic tales created for what they perceive to be a gentler female audience. Both men and women are feature directors, with style and intention all over the spectrum.

Smart Girl's Porn Vocabulary

Gonzo: A porn genre where there's no plot and the person with the camera directs the action, occasionally getting involved and giving the viewer a first-person experience. Takes its name from Hunter S. Thompson's irreverent, improvised situational style of journalism.

Hentai: Explicit, animated Japanese porn that typically includes use of taboo subjects such as sibling incest, transsexual sex, or sex with animals or with supernatural monsters, gods, and ghosts.

Lesbian, Girl–Girl, or All-Girl: In mainstream porn, a film that's all women, though the women performing are seldom lesbians.

Pro-Am: Short for "professional/amateur," describing participants who are new to adult films having sex with professionals, but can also include women who aren't really new to adult but are having a first-time experience on camera, or are experienced in adult but are new to a series. These films are all-sex, no plot, sometimes shot gonzo-style.

Specialty Porn: When porn's labeled "specialty," it usually contains a sex act or falls into a category outside conventional heterosexual tastes   though that can cover ground that many find disturbing or even shocking. Sometimes S/M is lumped into this category. Specialty can include transsexuals; fat folks, the elderly, or midgets; fetishes such as foot, breast, panties, or lactation; pregnant women; hairy women; and more.

Wall-to-Wall: These videos are all-sex, no-plot. They're usually a tape of sex scenes strung together loosely by a theme, like amateurs, or focusing on a sex act, such as fellatio, or both, as in first-time anal sex.

Gay Male

The vast world of gay male porn has a whole set of its own sub-genres, such as all-sex, plot-driven, bears (big hairy men), twinks (young-looking waifs), European (usually Eastern European), gay and bi (gay men with a woman thrown in the middle), S/M, leather, oral, pissing and fisting, romance, coerced sex, military, locker-room, interracial, and more. Gay male videos make up a whole, huge subculture and a thriving video industry unto itself, with many thousands of videos and subgenres for the viewer's pleasure. For girls who get turned on by watching men have sex, gay videos are the place to see men behaving sexually in ways that straight porn never shows, genuinely enjoying their own (and each others' bodies), and having sex with pure, unfettered lust. The way the performers react to each other is unlike the exchanges you'll see in straight porn; in straight porn you seldom see eroticism of the male body—men aren't intentionally the primary sexual focus.

For women who like to have sex with men, or who simply get turned on by male sexuality, this is a glaring omission in terms of what gets us off. Gay porn can fill this void by portraying a man-to-man exchange that can be simultaneously hot, hard, unforgiving, and tender. Many women find it a complete turn-on to watch the beefcake, heavily hung, sexually supercharged porn studs give and get as much as they can take, and find there's a lot to be learned about male sexuality from watching gay porn—much more than what barely bubbles to the surface in straight porn. Additionally, I can't count the number of times I've heard straight women exclaim, over the gay video box covers, how much sexier and more attractive the men in gay porn look than do straight male performers. Plus, man-on-man sex is just plain hot, perhaps in the same way as girl–girl scenes are for straight men.

The gay porn industry is huge and wide-ranging, comparable to the size of the straight-porn industry. Many gay-porn categories cater to dozens of very specific preferences (with themes such as facial come shots, young meat, big balls, huge loads, beefcake, Latinos or Asians or African Americans, orgies, sports and jocks, bears and cubs), whole series devoted to fetishes, and a subgenre of plot-driven feature films, each with its own favorite director. The budgets range from high to one-guy-with-one-camera low, the themes from loving to unbelievably rough, and the men from smooth-young-boy-types to older, big, hairy bears. But usually what you'll see in today's gay porn is similar to straight porn's overly groomed cult of hairless youth in the form of muscle-bound beefcakes—a big departure form 1970s gay porn when, as in the Golden Age Classics of straight porn, everyone had lots of body hair or a mustache, and didn't have a waxed chest, hairless balls, a gym-sculpted body, and a perfect tan line.

All-Sex, No Plot: Wall-to-Wall, Gonzo, and Pro-Am

All-sex films capture hot, one-time-only sex while it's really happening, with unscripted performances that show you what actually took place. The sex can be deliciously concentrated: thigh-shaking, white-knuckle rides through real female orgasms, chemistry that will have you picking your jaw up off the floor— and you're right there for every tasty minute. No bad acting, no plot to distract you. All-sex films are exactly that: all sex, with no distractions like acting, believability, sets, or frills. Most all-sex videos, especially the gonzo variety, are the reality TV of porn.

Videos with no plot and wall-to-wall sex are the ultimate instant-gratification visual sex toy. People who don't care about story line or characterization can cut right to the chase and get exactly what they're looking for—graphic sex and nothing else. These videos sandwich one tasty sex scene after another, making them suitable for repeat use, like a favorite sex toy. The viewer can play one scene, stop the DVD, and come back to try out the next scene later without feeling compelled to finish the story—and each new scene can be like a treat that you enjoy privately, just for yourself or with your honey. And if you find a favorite scene that bears repeat masturbation use, you won't have to guess about its location in the video. You can just skip to the scene or time marker, and replay your fantasy until you're spent.

All-sex films often suggest a theme that knits together a DVD or a series, and the individual scenes may be strung over a scenario or have a hint of fantasy elements. Such themes can be a viewer fantasy, such as voyeurism, in which case the camera-man sets up the scene as if watching through a window, from behind bushes, or from the perspective of a taxicab driver watching his fare in the rearview mirror. A theme can be the first-time performance of an actor, having sex with other performers, the cameraman, or solo. Or it can be the sex act itself: oral sex, multiple male partners, couples. All-sex videos can focus on a particular female performer, such as the *Deep Inside* series, where the actress introduces her favorite scenes. Or they can be compilations of scenes from other videos. You can find any one thing that turns you on in all-sex videos, and lots of it, exclusively.

Gonzo porn is also all sex, but filmed in a *cinema verité* style of candid realism. By the end of the 1980s, porn makers didn't need a big budget to make porn—just a camera. It seemed no longer necessary, and not at all practical, to create high-quality adult films like those that had screened in theaters. So in 1989 a new genre was born: gonzo, where the person with the camera directs the live and unscripted action, now and then also interacting with the performers. So-called after the improvised style of situational journalism popularized by Hunter S. Thompson, the genre elevated voyeurism into a style of video production. John Stagliano (aka "Buttman") and Ed Powers pioneered gonzo and are considered by many to be at the top of the trade, though they now share the field with talented contemporaries such as filmmakers Adam Glasser (Seymore Butts) and Britain's Ben Dover.

Gonzo often uses amateurs, whose enthusiasm and freshness can be arresting. Pro-am videos (for "professional amateur") depict participants who are new to adult film or who may be having sex with professionals for the first time. The genre also includes solo women in their first on-camera experience. The videos are all sex, often with a loose theme, and the quality varies widely. You'll come across videos with hot newcomers having amazing sex, as well as people who obviously aren't newcomers at all (but having great sex, too). You'll also find bored and boring actors, or experienced "newcomers" faking it badly.

Lesbian, Girl-Girl, and All-Girl

Guess what? The women in mainstream porn who make videos with *lesbian* in the title are rarely lesbians. Surprised? I hope you also don't believe in the tooth fairy. In fact, they're porn stars who "work with women," though occasionally they're bisexual in real life, and from time to time they turn out to be real lesbians. That's why *girl–girl* and *all-girl* are more appropriate words for their titles, and when you see a real lesbian film as opposed to a girl–girl video, you'll see the difference right away. Plenty of terrific all-girl porn exists on the market, in series like *No Man's Land* and *Screaming Orgasms*, featuring porn actresses who clearly enjoy going to work in the morning. But very few actual lesbian porn films include the whole spectrum of lesbian sexuality. And the real lesbian films are quite popular, with more and more coming on the market each year. You'll find them among features, all-sex, S/M, and other subgenres. But it's important to understand the difference between lesbian and girl–girl when you want to find porn that features women simply having sex together for fun, or women having sex who are actually lesbians. The real world's terms, and the real world's sex practices, don't exactly jibe with how the adult industry labels these things—so knowing the difference will help you make the selection you want.

Every standard straight, or heterosexual, adult video contains an obligatory girl–girl scene—a scene in which two or more of the starlets have sex. Most of the women who do the scenes are not considered lesbian, by either the industry or themselves, and certainly not by "real" lesbians. It's clear that these women are working and are lesbian for pay. When the makers of porn saw a gold mine for turning these obligatory scenes into full-length films, they created the "all-girl" market, marketing the porn as lesbian, though they well knew that the likelihood of these films having an actual lesbian in them was slim to none.

That's why real lesbians started making their own porn—even though lesbians enjoy girl–girl porn. Because they simply like to watch porn, they want to see the real thing, and women onscreen with whom they can identify.

Still, no one's really complaining here about watching two straight girls fuck each other. For me, it's like watching a guy who's gay for pay in gay porn; while he may be frowned upon in more politically correct circles, I really enjoy watching straight boys have sex with other men. And watching two women together is a powerful aphrodisiac, make no mistake. The all-girl videos show us an arousing side of female sexuality, and though many assume a male viewer, their women performers seem to relax more with each other without a guy in the scene. Some girl performers even regard bringing each other to orgasm as a game—and what a juicy game for two starlets to play! A good all-girl tape will have you absolutely glued to the screen, as you watch two women tell each other exactly how to make them both come—and then do it. If you're turned on by sex between women, it's as if a bolt of lightning hit your libido.

Real lesbian porn, by contrast, is where you'll see not only actual lesbians, but also a spectrum of female sexuality so diverse and powerful that you'll be blown away. And probably get pretty turned on, too, because it's tough not to become aroused watching what you know is sex purely for the participants, rather than an act that, by definition, is staged. Porn made by and for lesbians is not for people who want to see bodies by Mattel, so consider yourself warned. In these videos you'll see all body shapes and sizes, hair or no hair, femmes and butches, women wearing strap-ons who exude masculinity, tattoos and piercings and virginal skin, and rarely a boob job. A totally different standard of beauty is at play here, and a different standard of sex, too. You're guaranteed an authentic female orgasm in every scene, and furthermore these women have styles and methods of getting off that can't be matched by the adult industry, with its formulas and scripts. Not to mention that most of the real lesbian films often feature real-life lovers.

How Many Categories Can There Possibly Be?

Retailers and websites want to direct customers to their chosen category of porn as fast as possible, yet the result is a million crazy classifications, from the vague "straight" all the way down to "hairy all-girl underwater naked midget battles to the death." Okay, I made that one up, but you get the idea. And yes, many of the categories will shock and offend, confuse or arouse, and promise the impossible.

Here's a sampling from the website talkingblue.com: Adult Mainstream, Amateur Sex, Anal Queens, Animation, Asian Sex, Big Boob Babes, Black Erotica, Body Builders, Cat Fighting, Classics on Film, Compilations, Couples, Deep Throating, Double Penetration, Español, Euro, Facials, Fat Femme Fatales, Freaky Sex, Gang Bangers, Gonzo, Hairy Humpers, Incest, Interracial, Itty Bitty Titties, Latin Lovers, Leather and Lace, Lesbians, Lingerie, Mature, Midget Movies, Oral, Orgy, Parodies, Satanic Erotica, Sex Education, Shaving, Solo, Strap-on Babes, Strippers, Swingers, Tasteful Toes, Threesome, Vintage Voyeurism, Weird Sex, Wet and Messy, White House Sex.

S/M

S/M is a blanket term for sadomasochism; bondage and discipline (B/D); role-playing; and dominance and submission (D/S)—and nowhere is the term S/M more of a blanket than in porn of that genre. Such videos can cover all this ground (and more) within a single DVD, giving the viewer a front-seat ride through whippings, spankings, and hot wax treatments; exquisite Japanese rope restraints that look like works of art; women dressed as nurses or cops doing unspeakable things; and men who will do anything to please their mistresses. You can see outrageous—and extremely expensive—rubber and leather outfits adorning stern and beautiful dominatrixes, or skintight latex wrapped around the curvy asses of doe-eyed submissives. Some of the most-skilled experts in S/M can be seen using the poise and techniques that make them so good at what they do, and in many how-to videos on the market pros like these show you how to try S/M at home, safely.

But much of what you'll find here is eye candy, gas for the flames of your own fantasies and scenarios. Need an idea for an evening of pleasurably torturing the one you love? Pick up a Nina Hartley S/M how-to video, which mixes instruction with scenes designed to get your creative juices—and other juices— flowing. An S/M video can introduce a new idea into your relationship, perhaps opening up channels of communication that can take you closer to making your fantasies reality. Or perhaps you already enjoy S/M and just want some additional stimulation or masturbatory material that speaks to your personal preferences. Or maybe you simply think that women in fetish gear look hot. It's all here, in the world of S/M videos.

There are, however, a few things missing from S/M videos. For one, S/M videos suffer from many of the same complaints lodged against other porn features—technical problems like bad sound or lighting, ditzy porn stars with their "perfect" looks, and porn's minefield of unenthusiastic performers. A good S/M video will have high production values *and* look like a visual feat for the eyes—because, among other things, S/M is so very visu-ally arousing. A good video will show people who *look* like real people: sexy, sex-loving, and sexually alive in their everyday bodies (S/M films typically include amateur performers). And a great S/M feature will have players who are skilled, and whose chemistry and lust for each other make you sit up in bed and cry, "yes, Mistress!" while your hand sneaks its way into your lap. But still, something's missing from all S/M films, something that makes each and every one of these films unrealistic: no S/M video features sex. Read why in chapter 4, Why Porn Sucks.

Specialty

When porn is labeled *specialty*, it usually depicts a sex act or interest that falls outside conventional heterosexual tastes and might cover ground that some find shocking—or laughably familiar. This industry-labeled category lumps together bukkake, transsexuals, fat folks, elderly (sometimes geriatric), fetishes (such as foot, breast, panties, lactation, pregnant women, hairy women), and more. For some readers this may seem like a bizarre cabinet of sexual curiosities, but for others it provides a place where they can find what they want (albeit marginalized and usually badly made). Thrown into the specialty category is the category of extreme porn: videos that combine sex with themes or activities that are intended to shock or disgust the viewer.

chapter 7

not just for geek girls: online porn

O ne of the things I love the most about working on porn and sex blogs, besides getting to look at people having sex, is taking the porn I find and presenting it in context: smut for the sake of titillation, no shame, possibly with a hint of sardonic wit, criticism, and erotic sophistication. No matter what things I see and write about, the world of people will always involve sex, and nowhere is that more playfully exciting than online: something for every taste exists somewhere—for free. And if it's done well, and worth a click, it gets my good review— and if it sucks, then webmasters learn very quickly, from me and other critics, that they don't survive very long.

With online porn, consumers can just leave and never return, moving on to the next, better version of what they dumped. After all, there are no Mafia-style distribution networks forcing viewers into narrow categories, like there is in the world of porn DVDs. Consumer choice, erotic sophistication, active critiques in online porn forums...these things seem light years away from the attitude about porn displayed by mainstream media, with its dated-feeling scare-tactic articles and news stories about the horrors of online porn, the evils of smut peddlers, and all the other pulse-quickening tactics used by sensationalists to make the online world of porn seem like much more than it is (usually for extra ratings or site traffic). Seeing the online world of sex entertainment for what it is makes all the Halloween-haunted-house-cheap-fright tactics of "family" organizations and conservative journalism seem silly and childish, and transparent at that.

The truth is, rather than worrying about the evils of a photo that turns you on, you're better off worrying about what things the news or family site you just visited installed perniciously on your computer while you read their tabloid-style rantings. More often than not, news and family sites, along with travel and prescription drug sites, are among the worst offenders when it comes to multiple cookie placement, pop-ups, on-exit refresh, and other slimy tactics usually associated with porn sites.

But just because you're viewing porn, whether photos or video clips, doesn't mean that you're not going to need to safeguard yourself and take a few necessary steps to surf safely. Safer sex practices for your PC? It's much more than that. You'll simply notice that once you learn how to surf more safely for your porn pursuits, the rest of your online travels will go a lot more smoothly from here on out.

How to Surf, Safely

It's all up to the browser. Internet Explorer, Safari, Netscape—none of the programs you surf the Web with are as safe as Mozilla's Firefox. No one wants a computer clogged with tracking or redirecting cookies, which report on your surfing habits to marketing agencies or send you somewhere you don't want to go when you try to leave a site. No girl wants to play "Space Invaders" with a blizzard of pop-up windows, whether they erupt on a pharmacy website or after an accidental click on a porn banner linking you to an unknown or disreputable site. Just because you want to get down and dirty with your laptop doesn't mean you don't deserve a clean, well-lighted place to enjoy yourself.

If you just don't want to change your old ways and absolutely have to stick with your favorite browser, be sure to visit the browser's website and download and install the latest security patches (follow their directions). Microsoft's Internet Explorer is the most vulnerable, but you can set your browser preferences to automatically check for new security and virus patches daily— which you'll especially want to do if you're on a PC rather than a Mac, regardless of your browser. Unlike Apple computers, PCs, though they are the most-owned computers, are the most vulnerable to attacks, hackers, and viruses, and they need extra care, regardless of your porn-surfing habits. So take the time to safeguard your PC; download and install Firefox and you'll already be ten times safer than the PC girl next door. This goes without saying for Microsoft Windows users, who should also pay a necessary visit to SpyChecker.com, which offers an ever-growing selection of free antivirus, anti–pop-up, and virus extractor tools. Mac users have been resting easier for decades, as their computers have better security, contain built-in firewall protection, and are significantly more resistant to viruses. Safari (Apple) and Opera Web browsers both come with a number of excellent security features, including a stellar pop-up blocker.

Sure, learning a whole new browser like Firefox might seem like a pain in a girl's ass, but it's entirely worth it, especially because the new browser's precautions make surfing everywhere on the Web safer. Firefox users, for example, are constantly creating new ways to combat the latest pop-up technologies and ads being created to sidestep even Safari's pop-up blockers. Firefox is open source, meaning that it's free, and it's also easy for people to create new plug-ins for, meaning that there'll always be something new and fun (and safer) that you can add to your browser.

A few reasons why Firefox is the safest for porn surfing from squarefree.com/pornzilla/why-firefox.html (visit this page to read even more):

- *Control*: Firefox blocks unrequested pop-ups and never allows web pages to create hard-to-close full-screen windows. Firefox gives you options to prevent websites from resizing and focusing windows.
- *Security*: Malicious websites can never install spyware without your permission. Wank in peace.
- *Privacy*: Everything you might want to clear in order to cover your tracks—cookies, cache, download history, history—is in one place in Options. Firefox even provides a "Clear All" button to clear all this information quickly.
- *Extensibility*: The Pornzilla bookmarklets and extensions can improve your porn-surfing experience far beyond what any browser vendor would dare.
- *Images*: Firefox has an image-rendering library called "libpr0n" and a cute, unofficial mascot named Firefox-ko.

Smart Girl's Online Porn Vocabulary

Bookmarklet: One-click tool that adds extra functions to a web browser; also called "favelets."

PuNIC: A Firefox browser extension that lets you hide porn quickly.

Pop-Up: When a website opens a new window without your consent upon visiting a page; usually contains an advertisement. Sometimes called a "pop-under," meaning behind the window. Browsers like Firefox and Safari allow you to block pop-ups, and other free programs do the same.

Pornzilla: Tools and add-ons for Firefox specifically related to porn surfing: www.squarefree.com/pornzilla.

TGP: Acronym for Thumbnail Gallery Post, a post in a blog or on a page with small pictures (thumbnails) that link to other galleries.

X: A Firefox browser extension that clears all your private data and covers your tracks.

Go Go Go, Pornzilla

Porn is frustrating for many reasons, but one of the biggies on the Web is efficiency—you're liable to waste lots of time and endure pointless clicks, dead ends, and moved (or disappeared) websites. I believe that porn surfing should be pleasant, enjoyable, and time well spent, which is one of the reasons I love Fleshbot.com so much (not just because I work there). But aside from porn blogs like Fleshbot that can point you safely toward content, you can tweak, tease, and spank Firefox into a mighty porn-delivery machine with the many extensions and bookmarklets from Pornzilla.

At Pornzilla (squarefree.com/pornzilla), the community of contributors deliver "porn surfing, redefined." They feature an ever-growing roster of bookmarklets, little add-ons for your bookmarks toolbar that can greatly enhance a girl's porn-viewing experience—and it's as easy as clicking on the bookmarklet, dragging it up to the browser toolbar, and it's all yours. For instance, there are bookmarklets that zoom in and out of images with a single click; remove redirects from thumbnail galleries (useful when a TGP—page linking to many thumbnail gallery posts—uses redirecting links that sometimes go to an advertiser instead of the gallery), hide visited links (useful for TGPs where it's hard to tell which galleries you've already visited), and more. I really like the Google.com bookmarklets that allow me to search for similar galleries without even touching my keyboard.

There are thousands of Firefox extensions, and there are many particularly excellent ones for porn surfing; Pornzilla has collected a nice list of several. These extensions are easy to download and offer a number of great options you might not have considered, such as PaNIC, which lets you hide porn quickly; "X," which is a toolbar button that clears private data; and other tools that let you download entire galleries or sites, or show only the first images from galleries before you click so you can decide if they're even interesting to you or not. Granted, some of these aren't for novices, but even if you don't care about galleries or don't know TGP from CNN, the privacy add-ons are valuable resources. Pornzilla also offers helpful guidelines for making Firefox even more bug- and irritation-proof, like investigating Firefox's "Options› Web Features› Advanced," which lets you control what web page scripts are allowed to do to your browser; you can change your settings to prevent websites from resizing windows (when a site makes the window really huge), raising windows (keeping its window in front of others), and disabling context menus (preventing your right-click or CTRL-click mouse options).

The Evils that Porn Sites Do

Is your computer acting weird? Do most of the sites you surf seem to have pop-ups, do you keep ending up on a "hot chick" site, is your computer running super-slow, or are you having trouble every time you try to log into Yahoo? You've been made a victim of the evils that porn sites do...and you'll need to clean up your computer and browser, then run some antivirus software to fix the problem.

Aside from pop-up window blizzards, there are a number of truly lame (and downright evil) things that sites can do while you surf, peaceably trying to have a nice wank like the nice, smart girl that you are. Some of those listed below can be side-stepped with a good browser or up-to-date security, but others are the hallmarks of irresponsible webmasters who should be blacklisted, taken to task, or at the very least seriously ignored, like really hard. And if you come across any of these problems when visiting a site through a reputable reference such as AskJolene.com, Fleshbot.com, or even Google.com, report their tactics and they'll likely get blacklisted and removed from search databases. And as I mentioned, these unethical practices aren't restricted to porn sites but can occur on any site desperate for your visit.

Window Resize: When a site makes the window really huge—so big that you can't resize the window yourself and have to close the whole thing to continue.

Raising Windows: The offending site's window (or ad) stays at the front of all your browser windows no matter what you do.

Disabling Context Menus: When you right-click or CTRL-click your mouse, you usually get a little menu with various options like "copy, paste, close window," etc. Some sites won't let you use these menus, so you can't close the window or other functions.

On-Exit Refresh: When you try to leave their site, they force you to visit their site again, or take you to one of their advertisers or affiliates.

Circle Jerk Linking: It's not as fun as it sounds—this is a site that looks like a link list or TGP, but all the links on the page are usually blind links to sponsors and to other sites. A circle jerk uses a special script (or program) that tracks the number of clicks that a webmaster sends to the circle jerk. Then it sends out a number of clicks equal to or greater than that number.

Disabling Visited URL: Usually when you visit a link, it turns a different color so you can see that you've already been there—this is a function of your browser. When it's disabled by a site, you can't tell you've already visited the URL and may be on a page with seemingly different site links that all lead back to the same website. Pathetic!

Redirect: This is when you click on a link and it takes you somewhere completely different, or reloads the page as you visit the address you thought you were visiting. It's an outright non-consensual lie, and a redirect will get a site blacklisted from Google.

Cheater, or Irrelevant Result of Search Query: This is all too common throughout the Web with non-porn sites, as many webmasters will place search terms along their site that have no relation to their content—but I'm sure you've seen search results that look like a string of nonsense with your search word embedded in it. This is a cheater and there's little to be done except not click on it, though if you find it in a porn search site like AskJolene.com report it immediately for black-listing.

Gallery Spyware or Virus Installs: True evil—sites or downloads that install viruses or software that infect your computer and/or track you and report your information to others. A virus is a rogue computer program, typically a short program designed to disperse copies of itself to other computers and disrupt their normal operations. It must be cleaned up with an antivirus program. Spyware sends information about your surfing habits to its website. Often quickly installed on your computer (unbeknownst to you) in combination with an enticing free download, spyware transmits information in the background as you surf. Also known as *parasite software, scumware, junkware,* and *thiefware,* spyware is occasionally installed just by visiting a site (called a "drive-by download"). Internet Explorer and Windows are the primary targets of these evils.

Dialers: Programs that use your connection (via a network, ISDN, or phone line) and use it to commit fraud, often at your expense. People with DSL or similar broadband (cable) connections usually aren't affected.

Browser Hijack: Part of spyware and virus installs—forces you to sites where you don't want to go.

Free Videos: Clip Sites and Torrents

It was once estimated that Silicone Valley, where porn is made, cranked out around 12,000 porn videos (full-length VHS or DVDs) each year; we can only imagine how much video continues to be produced, in addition to the thousands of porn sites on the Web. And on the Web, one of the best ways for porn people from all walks of life (movie makers, starlets, niche sites) to promote their content is with short video samples of their wares. Naturally, this leads to literally tens of thousands of free porn clips floating around out there in cyberspace, just waiting to be watched by *some* smart girl...

Of course, this never means that what's out there will be any good; so, just like with the criteria you'd use for selecting a DVD to watch at home, you'll need to be somewhat patient and discerning, and to keep your expectations in check. After all, we're not buying the cow here—but the milk, even if it's only in thirty- or sixty-second increments, is pretty sweet when it's free. Fortunately, there are a number of sites (always changing and increasing) that collect links to free clips as their exclusive service and offer them up in a variety of ways. My favorite has always been ClipHunter.com, which categorizes the clips and allows for you to report on bad webmasters. (Their sister site, PicHunter.com, collects free porn galleries.) At Fleshbot.com we review and rate these sites as well (search: "video"), and I also like LonelyBit.com, Blinkx Video Search (blinkx.tv), Pornolizer.org, Wongle.org, 1036 Nice Porn Videos (ultraz.dk), and AskJolene.com. The Smart Girls' Porn Club has recommended: empornium.us, sweetflix.com, al4a.com, thehun.com, ampland.com, sublime-movies.com, amateurhomevids.com, and privatepornmovies.com. There are also a growing number of blogs that post clips daily:

dixler.blogspot.com is a recommended favorite. Individual film and performer sites will have free porn clips as well, and the indies are a gold mine for hot free content—they know how to promote a product. Visit ComstockFilms.com, StellaFilms-Production.com, PinkGasm.com, and AnnaSpansDiary.com.

Torrents, or BitTorrent file sharing, are a way of sharing files where the files (usually large, like video) are broken down into smaller chunks for easy downloading and distributed among different users: when you're downloading a torrent you're also uploading it to another user simultaneously. This way, every-one shares in the bandwidth load, so to speak—kinda like group sex. To get detailed information about how this works, visit Brian's BitTorrent FAQ and Guide (dessent.net/btfaq), or Wikipedia.org and Answers.com—type in "BitTorrent." As with any technology, torrents are excellent for swapping, or sharing, porn files. You'll want to check out clients such as Shareaza at shareaza.sourceforge.net.

An ever-increasing number of torrent sites have porn sections, and some are exclusively devoted to porn swaps. A few recom-mended sites for torrent exploration are: Torrent Spy (torrentspy.com/directory.asp), Empornium.us, PureTNA.com, Gay-Torrents.net, GayTorrentNews.org, PornBits.net, Muff-torrent.com, Hardcore Torrents (guide.hardcoretorrents.com), and of course, visit the official BitTorrent site, torrent.com.

Video on Demand

If you have a favorite porn director, actress, or series title, chances are good that their parent company's website offers you the option of watching their releases from the comfort of your computer—for a fee, of course. A casual trip to sites such as Maria Beatty's (BleuProductions.com), Evil Angel (EvilAngel.com; "DivX"), or Falcon (FalconStudios.com; "FalconFlix") will render options for being able to rent or stream to your computer almost any video in their catalog. In the case of Maria Beatty's site, her videos are part of a giant database of many related videos; so if you wanted to watch one of her terrific indy lesbian S/M videos, you could also add on a little time with an explicit Shibari rope bondage video from Japan. Still other adult retail sites like Gamelink.com offer a wide inventory of videos from myriad makers.

The way these on-demand systems generally work is by streaming the video (they send it to your preferred player in a browser window), or by allowing you to download the video to your computer as a rental for a certain number of days, depending on how much you pay. Each rental is encoded with a time stamp that locks the video after your time is up and prevents using it anywhere other than your original computer. Rentals typically have the options of lasting one, seven, or thirty days.

The great thing about video on demand is that it lets you see new products and choose from an incredible variety of them—*far* more than your local video store or typical adult retailer could possibly offer. You can also see parts of videos relatively cheaply; many systems allow you to buy blocks of minutes, similar to a phone card, that you can spend in any way you like, on any video you want. You don't need to wait for a video to arrive in the mail or have to cough up $40 to $50 to see that fetish video that turns you on; watch it right now, for $3.49, no waiting.

But like any technology, nothing's perfect. Videos that stream to your browser window tend to hiccup or hitch, creating frustrating skips in the action; your bandwidth will decide how easily you can watch the video (broadband is usually required). There are often a limited number of hours you can watch the movie, even if you rent (download) it—anywhere from one to five hours. The videos play in either embedded players if you stream, or if you rent they play in Windows Media Player or Real Player. None of these systems are made for Apple operating systems, and while some will work just fine on WMP or Real, others (sadly, Evil Angel's, for instance) don't work with Mac, Linux, or any open-source operating systems—Gamelink.com's VoD won't work on Apple computers outright. Video on demand at aebn.net has the best selection, but works best on PCs, and only okay on Mac systems, though they are beginning to provide iPod-ready porn from a huge selection of companies. Many VoD companies require use of Internet Explorer for streaming—ironically, the least-secure browser. You also have to deal with system requirements, such as available memory and computer processing speed. All this, plus reading through the privacy statements and terms of use, is enough to ruin a girl's woody.

Free Galleries, Erotic Photography, Flickr, and Babelogs

Finding free erotic images on the Web isn't difficult, by any means, but narrowing down what you'd like to see and then finding it, is. There must be hundreds of thousands of still photos taken and posted on the Web every year, from the lowest-budget amateur porn and homegrown couples' hard core, all the way to highbrow fashion photographers getting down and dirty with models, and erotic artists of every stripe. It's a vibrant, fierce culture of celebratory sex, art, and just plain smut: a smart girl's paradise. Finding it is easier than you think. You can spend your time hacking away through a search engine like Google in a hit-and-miss search, or you can let sex bloggers, adult gallery sites, and other art sites do the searching for you.

Needless to say, I spend a lot of my time at Fleshbot.com finding these sites and posting them there; you'll get an endless supply of interesting, amusing, hot, and sometimes-hilarious wank content with each visit or archive search. Follow the links off Fleshbot and you'll discover even more sites that collect and feature erotic content, from the explicit to the artistic (and often both). Other sites strive to do the same and do it well; sexblo.gs is a Euro site devoted to sex and culture, with multitudinous links to various sites and wanky content; even their ads lead to reputable porn. Erotic photographers tend to put their work online for free, or at least a significant number of tasty teasers— sometimes enough to get the job done. These sites are easy enough to discover through the aforementioned blogs, and through sites like Art Nudes (artnudes.blogspot.com) and Flickr.com.

Flickr.com is an online photo community where people create galleries and photo journals, and categorize them with a system of "tags." A tag is a descriptive word associated with the subject of a photo, so if you went to their search area and typed in "cleavage" you'd get a random, recent sampling of shots that include cleavage—sometimes sexy, sometimes silly. Flickr doesn't contain porn per se, but a tasty photo can lead to a member's profile with a link to their website, thus leading to an adult site, or at least a great erotic photo collection, and possibly the discovery of a photographer or model (or couple) you might like. Many sites, like softr.blogspot.com, collect the Flickr photos they think are the sexiest and post several times a day—sometimes, nothing's better than letting other people's fingers do the walking!

Nowhere does the world of online porn become more mind-boggling (to me) than the ever-morphing landscape of babelogs. A *babelog* is a frequently updated blog that links to different networks of affiliate galleries or TGPs, usually featuring ten to twelve photos of one model, one photo session, or a theme. Babelogs are free, the galleries are free, and supposedly the affiliates make their money through conversions, click-throughs that supposedly deliver a paying customer every now and then. But what we get are lots of high-quality, high-resolution (read: big)

RSS or PMS?

Okay, so a blog is an online journal, but what's RSS? Basically, RSS (Really Simple Syndication) is when updated content, like blog entries, have a special code that allows certain software programs to "subscribe" to them. These programs are called aggregators, and many are free to download—though Web browsers like Safari and Firefox let you subscribe by clicking on a button in the browser window. By subscribing to a blog, online forum, or podcast, you automatically get the newest post or upload delivered to your aggregator. A lot of people like RSS because it's a really easy way to keep up with news of all types, and it's great for following sites that post infrequently. Many aggregators are customizable and allow you to determine specifically what you want to have delivered, and how often. SexbyRSS.com offers explicit feeds by genre and categories, while the cleverly named del.icio.us is an RSS porn goldmine.

photos of sexy women. They're almost always women, or women together, and most galleries feature explicit pinups, though every so often you'll come across a shoot with penetration, usually with sex toys or strap-ons. Some are boring, some are silly, some are unintentionally retro porn-feeling, most convey only feminized standards of beauty—though a great many feature some of the most beautiful, sexy women I've ever seen. Babelogs are a great place to find pictures of really sexy European women and unconventionally sexy models, photographed with erotic expertise. There are more babelogs than can possibly be listed here, but a few favorites are labatidora.net, amables.com, babes.coolios.net, and the woman-run sensuallib.com.

Podcasts

Audio erotica has come a long way—and if you're wondering about erotic podcasts and "porncasting," that's basically what it's all about. A podcast is an audio file (in MP3 format) that's recorded and then tagged with a special code that allows people with certain software (like Apple's iTunes) to listen, or subscribe, to the show. Like radio, it's free, but the similarities end there: literally anyone can make and distribute a podcast, there's no limitation on content, and it's a listener-driven market, meaning that consumers have a choice about what, who, when, how, and where they listen to a show. The media were quick to jump on the uncensored aspect of podcasting, calling sex podcasts "porn" before anyone understood what the medium was—surprising a large number of listeners who expected typical porn when they hit "download" but often got erotica, interviews with dominatrixes and porn stars, sex ed, and all kinds of sex entertainment of the audio variety. And that's just what you'll find when you search in iTunes, Podcast Alley, Odeo.com, or iPodder—plus a whole spectrum of quality from the sublime to the beneath contempt.

Porn hasn't been known for its substance in terms of content, so labeling adult podcasts as porn was superficial, to say the least. But with the rising popularity of video/MP3 players like the iPod Video and the ease in podcasting a video file (M4V), there's a plethora of iPod-ready porn, available from both amateurs and mainstream porn makers. So now, for what it's worth, you can get the same free samples as with clip sites and watch them on a teeny-tiny screen, or you can buy iPod-ready videos for the same teeny-tiny screen.

Make Your Own Erotic Slideshow

Porn is lacking, the music sucks...so why not just make your own? When cruising around the Web, you'll often find a picture here or there that flips that little arousal switch to "on." Sometimes you might even find entire, tasty galleries. And maybe you want to enjoy them for your own private use later, or possibly you want to make your own porn—something a gazillion times better than "White Trash Whores #57." How about taking that slideshow function in iPhoto and making a special triple-X show, just for you (and a friend)? Making an erotic slideshow with audio on your computer is easy and can be excellent for putting on in the background while you get busy with a lover... Or enjoy fun images of your choice while listening to a sex podcast or several! Warning to all delicate and sensitive PC-using readers: *this is a Mac porn tutorial.* But, take notes, because this DIY (do-it-yourself) porn slideshow project can be translated to Picasa (picasa.google.com). Some users like it better than iPhoto, claiming it's faster, has more editing options, and is still quite intuitive. Picasa has similar slideshow capabilities to iPhoto, though it lacks the convenient integration with iTunes for choosing music.

Step 1: Images
First off, I'm not telling anyone to take and use photos that don't belong to them. But I know that lots of people have caches of hot photos they love to visit when feeling amorous (or self-amorous) or stumble across an image that just begs to be in their private collection. Drag the image to your desktop or right-click to save it. Open iPhoto and drag the images into your library. Better yet, get out the digital camera and make your own naughty slideshow—then show it to (or give it to) your lover.

Step 2: Make a Dirty Slideshow
Select the pictures and click the "new slideshow" button at the window bottom. Now you're looking at your slideshow in the main window. Give it a name—but unlike porn box covers, you'll use spell-check, right? If the pictures aren't in the right sequence, you can drag and drop them into the order you find most pleasing. You can also add new ones by dragging more from your library or the desktop.

Step 3: Editing
Click on the "settings" button to tweak the duration, scale, fades, and music settings. This will give you a chance to make a long, languorous slideshow or a quick and dirty flip-through that goes right to the money shots. How do *you* prefer the transitions

between photos—does the hottie in the photoset strip for you in a fade, mosaic, dissolve, page flip, reveal...?

Step 4: Music
I can't even begin to relate how many times I've started watching a hot DVD and had the music completely ruin my arousal—bad music is one of the ultimate girly hard-on killers. Still, porn videos continue to have music that sucks so bad I'm considering going to a hypnotherapist to erase the psychic scars these experiences have left on my libido. But in iTunes, you can add any music you want to your private porn slideshow, or a dirty podcast if you want hot talk (or no music at all). Click the "music" button at the bottom of the window to bring up your iTunes library and make your selection. If you want to use more than one song (or podcast), select a playlist. Once you've made your selection, go back to "settings" and "fit slideshow to music." Know that if you loop the slideshow, the pictures will drift out of time with the audio.

Step 5: Enjoy!
This may not be what iPhoto was made for, but it sure is a fabulous sex toy—slideshows can be used solo or coupled, or even with a group. Imagine lighting candles and having your hot production with its sexy music run in the background while you exchange erotic backrubs with your hottie du jour. (Sexy slideshow + Portishead + warm massage oil = sublime.) Or, maybe you'll find it a novel way to listen to your favorite erotica being read in a podcast. Don't forget that if you want to have the slideshow running for a while you'll need to go into your System Preferences and change your screen saver and sleep settings, so

your computer doesn't time out before you do. Your slideshow can be exported as a QuickTime movie (for private use only, of course)—just go to "share" and hit "export" and select a size. Choose small sizes for emailing and large sizes for burning to a CD. Visit apple.com/ilife/iphoto/slideshows.html for more (unintentionally dirty) slideshow tips.

Sex Blogs and Porn RSS Link Fun

Just like body types, sex blogs come in varieties and styles too numerous to list, but the important thing to know is that the online journal has become the ultimate medium of free self-expression and democratic communication—and nowhere is this more evident than in the world of sex blogs. Couples from France having sex with multiple strangers, taking photos of their amours, then posting them; anonymous exhibitionists of every permutation; anguished fetishists detailing their exploits; bisexuals floridly, graphically describing their sexual adventures at sex parties, on Craigslist.com; sex news and porn gossip; bizarre Japanese fetish photo blogs; sex advice from respected sexologists and therapists; porn directors journaling their film-making experiences...all this and so much more. And it's all free, user-created, a cheap date, and available at the click of a mouse.

In fact, there's so much that it's overwhelming; that's why sites like sexblo.gs, del.icio.us, pornblo.gs, babelo.gs, Fleshbot.com, Kinja.com, ErosBlog.com, sexblogs.org, and Google's BlogSearch are invaluable in the constant quest for hot bloggy voyeurism. All aforementioned sites that end in ".gs" and ".us" have changed the way the Web uses tags, blogs, user-submitted online link collections, and porn with their various categorizing systems.

These sites have become a clearinghouse and virtual online phone book of porn sites grouped by tags, or category labels—and they've done it with the help of everyone else in the world.

To explain how this works, I'll use myself as a modest example. I created a simple user account at del.icio.us and put the "post del.icio.us" as a button I created on my toolbar. When I visit a site I want to save, or rather contribute, to the online pool, I click the button, write a little description if I feel like it, then I post it. It goes on my personal del.icio.us page, but also gets listed on individual pages bearing any tags I associated with it, as well as on various versions of del.icio.us.

So, when I click my toolbar button and post "Fleshbot.com," I give it the tags "sex" and "pr0n" (a spelling to remember, using a zero instead of a capital O, often used instead of the word "porn," theoretically to evade the censors). The link goes on my http://del.icio.us/violetblue page, but also on the http://del.icio.us/tag/sex page and the http://del.icio.us/tag/pr0n page. These tag pages are updated every time someone adds a link, making it an incredible resource for porn, sex news, and all kinds of other porn-related juicy Web tidbits. You don't need to have an account to visit the tag pages; you can bookmark them for frequent visits, or you can subscribe for updates with an RSS program. It's like a porn grab-bag; sometimes people try to post links for marketing purposes, but it's rare, and I often stumble on new porn, amazing erotic art, and strangeness enough to keep me entertained for hours. You can also see how many others have linked to the same link, and sometimes their individual pages yield great porn finds as well.

chapter 8

porn for couples

For many women, their first porn-watching experience is with a sweetheart, and if it's enjoyable at all, it's *really* enjoyable. Before you even start the DVD, the air is charged with the foreknowledge that you're both about to do something naughty, fun, and highly sexual together. That's a huge turn-on for many couples. Lots of couples like the whole ritual of renting (or buying) a DVD, setting the scene, and watching together—it's a powerful aphrodisiac for two.

When you pick something that you both are excited about, you each may have your own ideas about what you expect to happen—or what you *hope* to happen. Mostly sex, but how that sex happens is up to your individual desires. You might want to just use porn as a little inspiration, to get turned on and have sex while you watch.

One or both of you might have specific ideas about how the sex might progress, such as acting out what happens onscreen. He might hope you'll go down on him while he watches, and you might want him to do the same to you. And there's no reason you can't do both! One of you might have had in mind a particular sex act that you've hoped will be introduced into your sex life—then, by happy accident, you see it in the video! If this is you, then don't just sit there—make your desires heard. Your lover isn't a mind reader, and though porn is possibly the best conversation starter about sex, you'll have to indicate verbally at some point that you like what you see and want to try it yourself.

How to Talk About Porn with a Lover

When it comes to couples watching porn together, chances are high that one of you has the idea first, and must introduce the idea into the relationship. Some people are lucky and find their lovers equally curious about the possible aphrodisiac effects of porn on their shared sex life, and they look forward to trying something new that could really spice things up. Many who are introducing this new idea to a novice porn viewer will receive a mixed reply—part curiosity, part apprehension. A few folks will be met with a reluctance to talk about it, while others might meet an outright refusal.

Either way, for you to explore the idea together, one of you has to initiate the conversation—easy if you talk about sex and experimentation regularly in your relationship, daunting if you never talk about sex or porn. Not everyone has seen porn before, so it's possible that you're reading this book wanting to watch porn with a lover for your—or their—first time. Also, a significant number of people have watched porn and *not* enjoyed it, and they're apprehensive about trying again—unaware that there are literally hundreds of different types of porn.

If you've never brought up the subject of sex with your part-ner, don't worry. If you have what you consider a routine style of sex, telling your partner that you want something to change is scary, and starting a conversation about your desires to watch porn might make you feel extremely vulnerable—especially if you already watch porn on your own or used to watch it before your current relationship. Even more so if the kind of porn you like isn't politically correct. Opening yourself up and asking for something you want sexually takes courage and also gives you an opportunity to learn more about what your lover likes and dislikes. Your lover may wonder if you've had sexual secrets all along. But it's very likely that your opening up this deliciously erotic Pandora's box will give them the opportunity to tell you what's on their mind about sex, too.

Before you begin, think about how you might bring up the subject in a way that would feel safe for you: You might feel more comfortable renting a mainstream movie with a slightly explicit sex scene in it (some suggestions are on page 50) and comment-ing on the scene. Or do you think you'd feel okay asking your partner what they think about porn while you're entwined in an intimate cuddle? Another technique you can try is telling them you want to confess a fantasy—a sexual one—and that he isn't to reply right away. Tell them that you can have a conversation about it later; this gives both of you time to let the idea settle.

Consider ways in which you can encourage your partner to hear you out, and ask them to suspend judgment until you can explain why this is important, and how good this new sexual behavior is going to make you both feel—and be sure to reas-sure them that you find them incredibly sexy. The most important thing to think through beforehand is how you're going to make your partner feel safe when talking about it. Rehearse in your mind what you'd like to say before you actually have the conversation. Think through possible scenarios and imagine how they might react, so that you'll be prepared to flow with whichever route the discussion might take.

Watching Together

Introducing your partner to porn can be fun, and once you've come to the decision to watch together you have many fun ways to get the party started. The limits are your imagination, but here are a few suggestions:

- Together, look at a website with porn reviews or a porn rental site. It's a huge turn-on, and you can make a hot shopping list together.
- Venture together into the adult rental section of your local video store or a store that exclusively carries adult products. You don't have to get anything the first time out, but you can if it excites you.
- If you both find something that you think might be fun, make a date, complete with dressing up and making a whole night of it. This can be a good way to deemphasize the viewing—helpful for nervous partners while downplaying the effects of a potentially disappointing film.
- With a DVD you both want to watch, make a special surprise out of it. Mail it to them with a love note indicating a date to watch together, or slip it under their pillow, or wrap it up and present it as dessert after a romantic dinner.

Sex While You Watch

You can have sex in a variety of ways as the DVD plays, or not have sex at all and save your excitement for later. Here are suggestions:

- Try out the positions of the actors onscreen, following along with the action.
- Use positions that make watching easy for both of you. Try a reverse lap straddle ("reverse cowgirl"), or spooning facing the TV or monitor, or lying face-to-face but facing the screen. Bring your laptop to bed!
- Doggie-style works well if you have enough room. Incorporate extra furniture as props for comfort or easing injuries and mobility issues. A hassock or padded footstool can make doggie-style effortless for the recipient.
- Take turns watching the DVD while one person performs oral sex on the other.
- Watch with your hands in each other's laps under a blanket.

One alternative is to view the film in its entirety and have sex afterward. More than one couple I surveyed for this book claimed that after they watched porn that both parties thought was awful or boring, they had supercharged sex when the TV was off. Perhaps they were stimulated by explicit images, period, or felt like they had to show each other what genuinely hot sex was really like!

You don't have to be entirely consumed by the movie to use it to enhance your sex life. Instead of using the film as the main focus, use it as a prop or tool:

- Try playing a DVD for your lover to watch in one room as you dress (or undress) for sex in the next room—talk about getting ready!
- Have a video running in the background with the sound off for extra visual stimulation as you seduce your lover with a lap dance or massage.
- Be watching the video when they get home from work and pretend to be "caught in the act."

Couples who enjoy more-advanced sex styles, such as BDSM or role-playing, can use porn to their advantage in a number of ways. Folks who are used to employing negotiation, consent, and all the highly creative trappings of power-play in their sexual relationships will already have an arsenal of ideas about how to use virtually anything to torture and titillate their lovers, though here I offer a few ideas as well:

- If you're dominant, tie your (willing) lover to a chair where they "must" watch the movie. You can also instruct your partner not to move or speak...or else.
- While your partner watches a video, have your way with them. Use your lover as a sex toy while you enjoy the video.
- With bondage, the restrained party can be erotically tortured while the film runs, heightening their arousal.
- Have your partner view an entire video without being allowed to touch himself or herself.
- Tell your partner the movie the two of you are about to watch is what will happen when the DVD is over. Then do it.
- Comfortably watch and enjoy the film as your partner "services" you.

- If you both like to switch roles, one can be tied down to watch the video as the other orally services the bound participant.
- If you enjoy S/M, you can add to the feel of your "dungeon" by having an S/M video running in the background for ambiance as you enact your own scene.
- Role-playing along with the DVD is a lot of fun. Maybe your honey is a bad boy like the one in the video!

Porn Sex Games

Watching porn together is fun all on its own, but since variation is the spice of life, try any of these porny sex games to turn up the heat.

Any Game Will Do

The next time you play pinball, Ping-Pong, horseshoes, golf, poker, or any other game, make it the hottest you've ever played, with these sexy high stakes:

- *Secret Shopper:* The winner gets to select a DVD to watch together.
- *Be My Porn Star:* The loser must act out the winner's favorite scene from an adult video while the video runs.
- *Remote Control:* One wins control of the remote for the duration of a sex scene, or an entire DVD.
- *Watch Me Watch You:* The winner faces the screen, the other player faces away from the screen watching the partner. A swivel chair doubles the fun. Being tied to the chair is even more fun.

- *Bound Bliss:* One is tied to a chair and made to watch porn, while the winner has free hands to roam and enjoy their own body—and every inch of their bound subject.
- *Sex Toy Tease:* The winner gets a sex toy while the other is forbidden to use their hands. Then switch.
- *Surprise Buzz:* Using remote-controlled vibrating panties, a butt plug, or even simply a vibrator with a long cord, the winner controls the other's vibration according to their whims.

Give Me a Kiss

This game is similar to movie "drinking games" where everyone imbibes an alcoholic beverage in response to a repetitive onscreen activity—but this game intoxicates only your libido. Every time an actor onscreen says, "oh god," "oh yeah," "fuck, yeah," "yeah yeah yeah," or whines like a hurt animal, the fastest one to repeat the sounds gets to kiss the other one anywhere— or directs the slowpoke to kiss them anywhere they please.

Variation: The slow one must sexually mimic whatever the actor's counterpart is doing onscreen.

S/M Variation: When the dialogue is spoken onscreen, the dominant partner gets to pinch, spank, bite, or clamp a clothespin on the submissive—as the intensity of the dialogue increases, so does the pain (and both parties' pleasure).

My Favorite Chair

Talk about a thrill ride! Flip a coin before the video starts (this works best with an all-sex film). "Heads" gets to be the chair first. The other one sits on the "chair," and the "chair" is free to explore the sitter while the sitter enjoys the video. Switch at each scene.

Head of the Class

This one requires unheard-of self-restraint, but the results are well worth the wait. Watch an entire video without touching yourselves or each other. When the video is over, write down a list of your favorite parts or things you wish you had seen in it, then trade lists for later play.

Variation: You can watch the video on your own time and then slip the report to your lover in public, or someplace where doing so is naughty.

Selecting a DVD for Your Lover

Renting or buying a DVD for someone else isn't easy, unless you know the person quite well and have an intuitive feel for their likes and dislikes. I can't count the number of times I've had a friend tell me to go see a movie in the theaters, or lend me a copy of their favorite Hollywood film to watch, and been utterly disappointed or outright confused that the person I thought was my really smart friend would like such crap. But I shrug it off and think to each his own, and thank my friend anyway. And then I never borrow a movie from them again. This situation is even more acute when it comes to porn.

With porn, you're seeking to suit not only your lover's tastes in film, but also the whole complex world of their sexual likes and dislikes. Unless you know for sure that your partner likes films by Seymore Butts or videos with Rocco in them, you're playing a guessing game in which you need to be part detective and part intuitive sleuth. If you put some thought and research into your selections, the rewards will be many.

Your first step is to familiarize yourself with porn. Learn the subgenres and the context in which the sex acts are presented. Then think about what your lover likes and dislikes in movies, sex, and body types. Reflect on any comments you might have heard them say about porn, how actresses and actors look, or porn in general. Does this person think fake boobs are icky? Do they like it when sex is depicted roughly, or not rough at all, or very softly? Do they really like a particular sex act, such as anal sex or blow jobs? Have you heard them mention that they would like to watch porn, if only it were like a regular Hollywood film?

Cultivate an idea of what you think this person might enjoy before you shop, and make a list of prospective titles or types of porn. Ideally, the best thing to do is to go to a store or browse a website along with the person with whom you're going to watch porn. But if it's a gift, a surprise, or a planned event in which you're the lucky courier, consider renting or buying more than one title. Renting is the ideal scenario, because if you get something they don't like you're not out $30 to $50. This isn't an option for everyone, though many websites do rent porn online. Make your big leap together into the world of explicit onscreen sex a hot, fun-filled adventure—together!

chapter 9

porn resources for smart girls

It's important to safeguard your privacy when surfing the Web. Shop at reputable stores; if you're not sure about their reputation, see whether they have online forums where you can garner customer feedback, check to see if they have actual brick-and-mortar stores (a sign of stability), and Google their URL and name to see what you can dig up. Check to see what their privacy policy is—if it's dodgy, shop elsewhere. See how they ship their products—is it discreet and do the DVDs come in plain packages? And finally, see how their products are presented: If they have offensive or misspelled product descriptions or sell products that are unsafe, or if they just seem a bit off, then they'll likely treat their customers with the same disdain. Do they have annoying pop-up windows? Skip 'em. Shop with businesses you like (vote with your credit card!), and if they have a section with educational material or a stated educational mission, even better.

Online Porn Shopping, U.S.

Adam and Eve: adameve.com

Andrew Blake: andrewblake.com

Babeland: babeland.com (retail stores in Seattle, New York, and Los Angeles)

Blowfish: blowfish.com

Cult Epics: cultepics.com

Early to Bed: early2bed.com (retail store in Chicago)

Eve's Garden: evesgarden.com (retail store in New York)

Evil Angel: evilangel.com

Good Vibrations: goodvibes.com (retail stores in San Francisco; Berkeley; and Brookline, Mass.)

Hustler Hollywood: hustlerhollywood.com (retail stores in West Hollywood; Gardena; San Diego; Monroe, Ohio; Cincinnati; Nashville; New Orleans; Lexington; and Fort Lauderdale)

JT's Stockroom: stockroom.com

Libida: libida.com

Pleasure Chest: thepleasurechest.com (retail stores in New York, Los Angeles, and Chicago)

Pleasure Place: pleasureplace.com (retail store in Washington, D.C.)

Purple Passion: purplepassion.com

Sinclair Institute: bettersex.com

Smitten Kitten: smittenkittenonline.com (retail store in Minneapolis)

Tulip: mytulip.com (retail store in Chicago)

A Woman's Touch: a-womans-touch.com (retail store in Madison)

Xandria: xandria.com

Online Porn Shopping, Canada

Come As You Are: comeasyouare.com (retail store in Toronto)

Good For Her: goodforher.com (retail store in Toronto)
Lovecraft: lovecraftsexshop.com
Venus Envy: venusenvy.ca (retail stores in Ottawa and Halifax)

Online Porn Shopping, U.K.

Ann Summers: annsummers.com
Blissbox: blissbox.com
Cliterati: cliteratishop.co.uk
Hustler Hollywood: husterlhollywood.co.uk
LoveHoney: lovehoney.co.uk
Taboo: taboo.co.uk
Tickled: tickledonline.com

Online Shopping, Australia and New Zealand

Bliss for Women: bliss4women.com (retail store in Melbourne)
Femplay: femplay.com.au
Ms. Naughty's For the Girls: msnaughty.com
Sharon Austen: sharonausten.com.au

Online Shopping, Europe

Blissbox: blissbox.com (sites for shipping to Netherlands, Germany, and Belgium)
Concorde Boutique: concorde.fr (retail store in Paris)
Demonia: demonia.com (retail store in Paris)
Fleshion: fleshion.com (France)
Sexou: sexou.com (France)
Voissa: voissa.com (France)

Indy Porn Creators

Alternative Worldz: alternativeworldz.com

Anna Span: AnnaSpansDiary.com

Black Mirror Productions: blackmirror.com

Burning Angel: burningangel.com

City of Flesh / Stella Films: stellafilmsproduction.com

Comstock Films: comstockfilms.com

The East Van Porn Collective: eastvanporncollective.org

Erocktavision: erocktavision.com

Fatale Media: fatalemedia.com

Joseph Kramer / School of Erotic Touch: eroticmassage.com

Kink Media: kink.com (home to RealFuckingCouples.com and FuckingMachines.com, among many others)

Libido Films: libidomag.com

Lust Films: lustfilms.com

Maria Beatty's Bleu Productions: bleuproductions.com

Pink and White Productions: pinkwhite.biz

Pinkgasm: pinkgasm.com

Pirate Booty Productions: profanepirate.com

Red Board Video: redboard.com

SIR Video: sirvideo.com

Online Rentals

AdultDVDEmpire.com

AEBN.net (video on demand)

BlueDoor.com

BushDVD.com

FlickSmart.com

Gamelink.com

GreenCine.com
SugarDVD.com
WantedList.com
XRentDVD.com

Online Porn Resources

Adult DVD Talk: adultdvdtalk.com (forums and reviews)

Adult Film Databse: adultfilmdatabase.com

Adult Video News (AVN): avn.com

Altporn: altporn.net

Amazon: amazon.com

AVNOnline: avnonline.com

Dude Tube: dudetube.blogspot.com

Erika Lust's Blog & Vlog: erikalust.blogspot.com

Fleshbot: fleshbot.com

Hidden Self Forums: hiddenself.com/forums

Jane's Guide: janesguide.com

Kara's Erotica For Women: karaslinks.com

Ms. Naughty's Blog: msnaughty.com/blog/index.html (also has links to porn reviews, porn for women links, video on demand, and more)

Porno 4 Women: porno4women.com

Search Extreme: searchextreme.com

Second Life: secondlife.com

Seska For Lovers: seska4lovers.com

Sexblo.gs

Sexuality.org

Stockroom's Kinkwire Forums: http://forum.stockroom.com

Techyum: techyum.com

TGP.com
Tiny Nibbles: tinynibbles.com
Tristan Taormino's Pucker Up: puckerup.com
Viviane's Sex Carnival: viviane212.blogspot.com

Free Video and Clip Sites

1036 Nice Porn Videos: ultraz.dk
al4a.com
AmateurHomeVids.com
Ampland.com
AskJolene.com
Blinkx Video Search: blinkx.tv
Cliphunter.com
dixler.blogspot.com
Empornium.us
LonelyBit.com
Pichunter.com
Pornolizer.org
PornReports.com/reviewers.htm
PrivatePornMovies.com
Sweetflix.com
SublimeMovies.com
TheHun.com
Wongle.org

Safe Porn Surfing Resources

BoingBoing's Guide to Defeating Censorware:
boingboing.net/censorroute.html

Bumpercar: freeverse.com/bumpercar2 (smart, parent-moder-
ated Web filter to keep kids away from porn)

Extended pop-up blocking:
beatnikpad.com/archives/2003/03/08/adblocking

Firefox: mozilla.com/firefox

Pornzilla: squarefree.com/pornzilla

Tiny Nibbles Safe Porn Surfing Guide:
tinynibbles.com/pornsurfing.htm

Why Firefox: squarefree.com/pornzilla/why-firefox.html

About the Author

VIOLET BLUE is a professional sex educator, sex columnist, female porn expert, pro-porn pundit, and contributor to Fleshbot.com and Metroblogging San Francisco. She is the editor of the *Best Women's Erotica* series, along with *Best Sex Writing 2005*, *Lips Like Sugar: Women's Erotic Fantasies*, *Sweet Life: Erotic Fantasies for Couples*, *Sweet Life 2*, and *Taboo: Forbidden Fantasies for Couples*. She is the author of *The Adventurous Couples Guide to Sex Toys*, *The Ultimate Guide to Adult Videos*, *The Ultimate Guide to Sexual Fantasy*, *The Ultimate Guide to Fellatio*, and *The Ultimate Guide to Cunnilingus*, the latter two of which have been translated into French, Spanish, and Russian. Blue has appeared on Playboy TV's *Sexcetera*, NPR, and CNN, and she has been featured in such publications as *Esquire*; *Cosmopolitan*; *O, The Oprah Magazine*; *Salon.com*, *Newsweek*, the *Wall Street Journal*; and *Wired*. Visit her at tinynibbles.com or listen to her podcast Open Source Sex.